LIVING
LIGHT

LIVING
LIGHT

THE ART OF USING LIGHT
FOR HEALTH AND HAPPINESS

KARL RYBERG

ENLIVEN BOOKS

—

ATRIA

New York   London   Toronto   Sydney   New Delhi

ENLIVEN™
ATRIA

An Imprint of Simon & Schuster, Inc.
1230 Avenue of the Americas
New York, NY 10020

First Enliven trade paperback edition February 2019

For information about special discounts for bulk purchases, please contact Simon &
Schuster Special Sales at 1-866-506-1949 or business@simonandschuster.com.

The Simon & Schuster Speakers Bureau can bring authors to your live event. For more
information or to book an event, contact the Simon & Schuster Speakers Bureau at
1-866-248-3049 or visit our website at www.simonspeakers.com.

Interior design by Suet Yee Chong
Title page photography by klms/Shutterstock, Inc.

Manufactured in the United States of America

10 9 8 7 6 5 4 3 2 1

Library of Congress Cataloging-in-Publication Data

Names: Ryberg, Karl, author.
Title: Living light : the art of using light for health and happiness / Karl Ryberg.
Other titles: Light your life.
Description: First Enliven trade paperback edition. | New York : Enliven Books, [2018] |
    "Originally published [as Light your life] in Great Britain in 2018 by Yellow Kite, an
    imprint of Hodder & Stoughton, an Hachette UK company"—Title verso. | Includes
    bibliographical references and index.
Identifiers: LCCN 2018038291 (print) | LCCN 2018052039 (ebook) | ISBN
    9781501169984 (eBook) | ISBN 9781501169960 (pbk.) | ISBN 9781501169984 (ebk.)
Subjects: LCSH: Phototherapy. | Light sources.
Classification: LCC RM837 (ebook) | LCC RM837 .R93 2018 (print) | DDC
    615.8/31—dc23
LC record available at https://lccn.loc.gov/2018038291

ISBN 978-1-5011-6996-0
ISBN 978-1-5011-6998-4 (ebook)

CONTENTS

MY PERSONAL
LIGHT JOURNEY

My fascination with light started when I was a young boy growing up in Sweden. Dad was a cubist painter and worked on large canvases, to which he applied shiny layers of smelly oil paint. His atelier had large windows, facing north, toward the sky, and they gave the whole room a quality of transparency; he was always stressing the necessity of good daylight to get the subtle gradations of color right. I loved to spend time in that spacious studio, and somehow became fascinated with the shimmering interaction of light and color. Eventually I made crude attempts at painting, and a whole new world opened up before my eyes.

As I looked into the interplay of light and color, I wanted to find out more about the nature of this visual magic. This journey led me to study architecture as a young man. But if I thought my studies would help me to understand and indeed to learn more about the wonders of natural light, I was mistaken. It was the 1960s, after all, and the architectural approach to light was blunt and practical, and focused on artificial light; electric lamps were technical commodities to be switched on and off without any further thought. The outflow of light was promptly measured in watts and lux, the building blocks of electric light, and even though we humans were the end users of these technical wonders, there was very little mention of how they might affect us, emotionally or biologically. It was simply something that architects, and indeed consumers, didn't think about at that time.

Those of us old enough to remember will understand that those were the days of frantic modernism, of looking forward to a bold future, a brave new world in which machines would swiftly solve most of our problems. Nature was shamelessly tamed or maimed, and fluctuating daylight was considered an erratic and uncontrollable nuisance, best barred from organized life. In my native Sweden, futuristic schools were built without any windows at all to create a generation of standardized and brave new kids. The thinking at the time was that steady artificial light would *enhance* the process of concentration, and that the separation of humans from the world would improve their intellectual performance—but the outcome was a complete disaster. My country started to churn out a generation of children with poor intellectual performance: until 2015, Sweden languished on the lower rungs of the educational ladder, with averages in science, mathematics, and reading lower than those for the Organization for Economic Co-operation and Development (OECD). The political explanations are many, but, in my view, they neglect the impact of one key factor: lighting.

However, it was my very nationality that fueled my interest in all things light. As we know, Swedes occupy an extreme climate zone with huge luminous contrasts between seasons. This puts a definite strain on our biology, and mood swings are part of the game for many of us. In summer we are bathed in continual light and the sun doesn't even bother to set. Migratory birds come all the way from Africa to lay their eggs and enjoy the extravagant luminosity, and we Swedes celebrate the festival of Midsummer with eating, dancing, and great celebration. Nordic winters are another story altogether, with long, dark nights and barely any daylight at all. The looming shadows hang on for months. Many of us northerners hibernate indoors and binge on sweet carbohydrates by cozy candlelight. Alcohol is imbibed for additional consolation. The winter blues are a stark reality as the life juices slowly wane away. In Sweden, much of the population eagerly awaits the light of spring to recharge their batteries. The situation is more or less the same in the subarctic regions of northern Canada and Russia.

After finishing my studies, I went to work as an architect in Australia and New Zealand, where the light conditions are vastly different from those in Scandinavia. The luminous effects on people were enormous, and my curiosity about the effects of natural light led me to study psychology and medicine to find out more.

As I wrote my thesis on light therapy, I kept coming across the name Rosenthal in scientific papers. His research was revolutionary and literally shed new light on an old problem. Every Scandinavian knew of the dreaded winter depression, but no real remedy had been found. Women, with their naturally keen color vision, were much more affected than men, but traditional medicine would turn a blind eye and treat it as a collective form of female hysteria. Not until 1984 did Dr. Norman Rosenthal understand what we now know to be seasonal affective disorder, or SAD for short. Under the influence of darkness, the brain will produce the sleep hormone melatonin. This ancient habit worked fine for our African ancestors, because they lived near the equator and their climate came with little seasonal variation, but you can imagine its impact on those of us who live in the

Northern Hemisphere. In winter we would be sleepy for months on end! Moving entire populations back to the equator is, of course, an impossibility, so Rosenthal came up with the bright idea of using strong light to simulate sunshine and to stimulate hormones to get the brain back in shape. Somehow, his optic trickery seemed to work.

This was groundbreaking news. At last, someone had proven a clear connection between the level of ambient light and our mental health. Having returned to Sweden, I continued my studies in psychology to gain a better understanding of light and its effects on the human mind. To help in funding my studies, I opened a light clinic in Stockholm offering treatments with the new method. I called it *monocrom*, meaning "single color," and over the years my small practice has developed as I have learned more about the transformative qualities of light.

Dr. Rosenthal had recommended using white electric light in large doses to imitate daylight. White rooms in all light clinics were flooded with several thousand lux and the patients were supposed to wear white, too. The visual effect was quite stunning, as you can imagine. However, at the time, the only available sources of sufficient power were large fluorescent tubes, and even though they were effective in improving my clients' moods, people were less enthusiastic about all that ugly glare.

As a compromise, I started wrapping the fluorescent tubes in colored filters to provide more pleasant visual treatments, and I discovered that the purer and more radiant the colors, the happier my clients would be. The most beautiful colors are known as *monochromatic*, and these gorgeous eye-catchers are found in rainbows and peacock feathers. *Monochromatic* in this sense means strictly one-colored as opposed to *polychromatic*, or many-colored. The pure hues are technically difficult to achieve, but, after some searching, I found highly selective filter coatings that could deliver super light to my clients. The therapeutic outcomes were stunning. Empirically, I found that monochromatic light delivered better results more efficiently, with many clients reporting great benefits, such as incredible lifts in their mood, and many cases of winter blues could be alleviated or totally avoided.

My work in light therapy was going well, but I knew that more could be done. Coincidentally, at this time, I read a fascinating article in an international scientific journal, mentioning a Russian professor at the Russian Academy of Sciences in Moscow, Tiina Karu. She was doing research on the cellular responses to monochromatic light and her results were nothing short of revolutionary. Many biological effects of colored mono-light were proven identical to those of the miraculous laser, which was used medically in Eastern Europe at the time. Brain tissue was shown to be particularly sensitive to laser radiation, and intellectual performance would improve. Diffused laser light could also induce rapid wound healing and regeneration of skin tissue. The wounds treated with laser left no scars, and this was a huge cosmetic success. The Hungarian professor Endre Mester made one of the key discoveries in this field, finding that low-level laser therapy (LLLT) produced great results for pain-related conditions such as osteoarthritis. The biological effects of strictly one-colored—or monochromatic—light are identical or even better than laser light. (For nonbiological purposes like engineering or physics, they are not identical at all.)

Fortunately, it was the time of glasnost in the former Soviet Union, and President Mikhail Gorbachev had initiated a program of cultural exchange that was exceptionally open-minded, so I wrote to Professor Karu and invited myself over as a guest student. Snail mail was the norm in those days, and the response took a long while, but eventually a kind letter of invitation arrived, and soon I was on board an Aeroflot plane bound for Moscow.

Professor Karu welcomed me to Russia and personally guided me around the laboratories. I was fascinated to see the large halls with high ceilings filled with glass cabinets containing hordes of transparent vials and glowing lasers. One of her key discoveries was that monochromatic light can repair damaged mitochondrial DNA, which is the very powerhouse of the living cell. This irradiation will extend the normal life span of the entire cell, but what was crucial was the purity of the color. We will look at the technical side of things in chapter 2, but, in short, I learned that biological laser effects could be replicated by the monochromatic light I was already using. I couldn't wait to get back and upgrade my therapeutic equipment so that I could replicate—albeit on a smaller scale—what Professor Karu was doing in the Soviet Union.

With the help of my team of technicians, a new generation of professional color projectors could now be manufactured. High-pressure xenon bulbs—the kind of bulbs normally found in cinema projectors—were needed as light sources, and the light parameters had to be accurately defined. The optics were quite complicated, and in the beginning brilliant failures were produced. Finally we got the technical details right and could at last present this modern version of light therapy to our clients, at this time presenting with a range of issues, including sleeplessness, insomnia, depression, and even infertility. Clients and colleagues alike were surprised at the capacity of the new projection methods to be beautiful, restful, and healing. As many of us know, happiness and beauty are extremely powerful healing factors—extending far beyond their famed placebo effects. They give hope to the heart and form the very basis of successful psychotherapy, but today we also know that joyous states of mind are linked to cell repair. In response to emotions of happiness, it has been discovered that the brain starts to produce powerful healing hormones like endorphins and oxytocin, which are released into the bloodstream. This will ultimately affect the entire body.

In the case of my work, the positive therapeutic results came as a boost to us all, and the almighty grapevine did the rest. Word started to spread about our glorious Nordic Light and we began exporting the equipment. It became really popular, and thousands of people experienced the healing effects of monolight. More photonic tools were added to the list, and I finally had to close my private clinic to meet the growing demand and to train new generations of light workers. Competent researchers were widely scattered, so an international network and association was established, the International Light Association. No university offered any systematic training in the enigmatic science of light therapy. It was definitely a fringe discipline, and accessible literature on the subject was largely lacking. Old books and articles had to be plowed through, and new books and articles had to be written. Everyone knew what light meant—but offering light therapy as a remedy for body and soul was not a widespread idea.

Which brings me to *Living Light* and what my work, distilled in this book, can do for you. It's true to say that not all of us suffer from SAD or from other ailments that might respond to light therapy; not all of us experience depression or stress, thankfully, but it is my belief that good-quality light in our daily lives is far more important than we might think. Thankfully, the research is beginning to emerge to support my long-held views, which is gratifying, of course, but also of immediate importance to you, the reader. Enjoying the precious resource that is natural light will add so much more to your life: it will boost your reserves of vitamin D, but it will also make you *feel* so much better. And gaining insights into the role of electric light—and in particular the blue light that now dominates our lives—will help you to minimize its negative effects.

Understanding how your eyes work to absorb natural light and to see will be fascinating, but it will also help you in practical ways. The eye yoga exercises in this book might strike you as being a bit "out there" at first, but they are fun, relaxing, and might just help to keep your eye muscles in tip-top shape.

Understanding how natural light works in architecture will help you to use it well in your own home, whether you've been lucky enough to build it yourself or are living in an older home—many gloomy décor problems that seem insurmountable are easily conquered with a little well-placed illumination. And eating a nice, balanced "light" diet will not only help you to maximize your vitamin and mineral intake, but will also keep you feeling healthy and vital. Finally, the "color gallery" in this book's appendix will help you to understand more about the magic of color and how important it is in all our lives.

Living Light is the culmination of many years of work. For me, it's the fulfillment of a life's dream to be able to share my passion for light with you—it's a cookbook of sorts for a happy and luminous life. This is where my part of the journey ends. The rest is for you to enjoy.

2

WHAT IS LIGHT AND WHY IS IT IMPORTANT?

Light is the first of painters. There is no object so foul
that intense light will not make beautiful.

—RALPH WALDO EMERSON

The history and science of light is a fascinating—and puzzling—subject, one that has kept scientists busy for more than two thousand years. Understanding what light is has intrigued many of the finest minds, and even today the borders of the subject keep expanding.

We'll look at the exciting time line of discoveries in light on page 16, but first, let's ask ourselves the question, Why does light matter? Now, this may seem obvious, but think about it: Look around you and see what could function without light. Your humble houseplants need light to photosynthesize; you need sunlight to get your skin to manufacture vitamin D; the solar panels on your roof need sunlight to heat water for your showers and central heating; more fundamentally, our biological processes are driven by light. The sun, that hot ball of fire that seems to hang in the sky, powers every single ecosystem on earth. Imagine what our world would be like without the sun. Plants would wither and die, depriving the animals that feed on them of valuable food, depriving us of our own food . . . and so on.

But other forms of light have their own powers, too. Flame was one of the great innovations in very early life: When humans discovered that fire had a practical use, they could cook what they hunted, keep warm, and keep animals at bay, and, very important, use fire to shape the tools that helped them in their daily lives. As humans became more sophisticated, they began to see firelight as something symbolic: a hypnotic warmth that signaled bedtime, that could pierce the darkness to create a feeling of safety. Light forms the basis of festivals all over the world, from Saint Lucia's Day in my own country of Sweden, to Diwali in the Hindu calendar, symbolizing the light of spiritual enlightenment, the banishing of evil. Christmas is a Victorian invention, of course, but it's no accident that it lights up the darkest time of the year.

And let's not forget other forms of natural light, those that come from the moon and stars. To our ancestors, the heavenly bodies were not only powerful light clocks that ruled all life on earth—they also served as divine companions. Pagan religions saw them as celestial and mysterious vagrants. The Greeks called them *planetos* and the Persians named them *calendars*. Primitive humans feared the absence of the heavenly lights and performed ritual sacrifices, pleading with them to come back. The light gods would then mercifully return every day or month and grant their shining presence. The stars were vital for navigation, nighttime guides for travelers wandering the globe.

In nature, the strong gravitational pull of the moon rules the tidal waters and influences all marine life. Our monthly calendar is based on the four phases of the moon, and it is thought that in some ancient way, tidal forces also coordinate human body fluids in general—the menstrual cycles of women can be linked to lunar phases, for example. The beams of a full moon are thought to have strong hypnotic qualities on both animals and humans: Dogs and wolves howl at the moon, and lunar cults celebrate their own rituals. One study on pet behavior and the moon "identified a significant increase in emergencies for dogs and cats on fuller moon days (waxing gibbous to waning gibbous), compared with all other days."[1]

Light controls many of our functions, but significantly, the contrast between the brightness of the day and the velvety darkness of the night is also of deep importance to humans and animals. How else can we function, but to tell night from day, when it is time to wake and time to sleep? A look at babies and their chaotic sleep patterns tells us that this process, called *entrainment*, isn't built-in, but is rather a matter of synchronizing our internal systems to the natural cycle of light and dark, a cycle that has been with us since the beginning of time.

Many of you will have heard of the term *chronobiology*, perhaps because of the three scientists who won the 2017 Nobel Prize for their study of circadian rhythms, Jeffrey C. Hall, Michael Rosbash, and Michael W. Young. In essence, every cell has its own inner clockwork mechanism, where ratios of cellular molecules pulsate back and forth in chemical oscillations. The semi-stable rhythms are called *circadian*: the Latin word means "circa one day." These rhythms literally float around, and the enormous numbers of loosely linked biological reactions need firm coordination or they will quickly create havoc, like a band of amateur musicians without a competent conductor. And the conductor of this cellular jam session, keeping trillions of reactions in sync? Our old friend the sun.

Sunlight fed through the eyes will signal a master chronometer, or timekeeper, located inside the brain, known as the suprachiasmatic nucleus (SCN). This group of neurons is triggered by incoming light and sets in train a host of bodily functions. What an extraordinary thing this is.

So light is an energetic and temporal marker that gives a definite pulse to the day—an organic body clock without hands. Levels of light and darkness have accurately programmed our biological systems to different modes of activity. The timing of daylight and starlight is the most basic of all biological rhythms. It will resolutely reset your body cycles to their default state and indicate when it is time to sleep and to work.

There have been a number of experiments to test the role of daylight in programming biological systems and what happens if the natural cycle of day and night is taken away. In 1964, two cave explorers, Josie Laures and Antoine Senni, were sent to live in deep caves near Nice, France, in an experiment to study the effects of isolation and light deprivation on humans. They were to live in separate caves, without any daylight or clocks, and their responses to their environments were communicated to scientists on the surface. When Laures emerged from her cave after eighty-eight days, on March 12, she had noted the date as February 25, while Senni, who spent 126 days underground, recorded periods of sleep as long as thirty hours, without having any real sense of time passing. Without natural daylight followed by night, both found that their sleep–wake cycles quickly became disorganized and their sense of time passing was completely disrupted. In a later experiment, in 1993, Maurizio Montalbini, an Italian sociologist, spent a total of 366 days underground in a cavern in Italy, but when he emerged, he had recorded only 219 days as having passed. But of even more interest was his new sleep–wake pattern: during a forty-eight-hour period, he would be awake for thirty-six hours and asleep for twelve. It is clear that without the natural cycle of day and night, the entrainment of our internal biological processes begins to fall apart.

And natural light has an effect on mood, too. A study on rats conducted at the University of Pennsylvania, which deprived the creatures of light for long periods of time, found that "the animals not only exhibited depressive behavior, but also suffered damage in brain regions known to be underactive in humans during depression."[2]

We also know now that light plays a crucial role in seasonal affective disorder (SAD). Interestingly, the appearance of SAD links back to the earliest humans, when hibernating to some degree was thought to be useful, particularly in pregnancy, which consumed energy. Some researchers believe that this "throwback" might explain why women suffer more from SAD than men. But research has also shown that lack of light in the wintertime has an impact on the part of the brain that produces serotonin, that mood regulator essential for our psychological well-being. (Some populations, notably Icelanders, have a gene that is thought to help them produce more serotonin to keep them going through the winter!)[3]

So we need natural light to function, and we also know that it plays a crucial role in the way our bodies work, but what happens when we introduce electric light into the equation?

Electricity is one of the great inventions of the modern era, powering many of the light innovations we take for granted. Imagine what an exotic oddity it was some hundred years ago! Hotels had to put up instructions to prevent innocent guests from trying to ignite the new light bulb with matches, and at bedtime confused visitors would still try to blow out the bulb like a candle. The earliest electric lamps were used for public lighting in large, open city spaces. Place de la Concorde was first: The Paris police wanted strong light to act as a deterrent to the rampant criminality of the day. The oldest electric home lighting systems were designed only a century or so ago and cost a small fortune to install, but you can imagine the difference it would have made to people: no glowing embers and no filthy ashes to carry around; no lethal fumes and no need for elaborate chimneys.

Of course, the advent of electric light—particularly its introduction to the masses in the Western world from the 1930s on—has changed the way we live. With the widespread use of electric light, we spend more time indoors in artificially lit environments and, crucially, spend more time at work. All progress, you might say, until you consider the impact of electric lighting on our ancient biological processes.

Many studies have shown that electric light, while a boon, affects the way we sleep. A 2013 study in *Current Biology*, in which a group of people were exposed to a week of camping in the great outdoors, without the aid of any kind of artificial light, followed by a week of the same activities, but this time with electric light, showed some very interesting results. "Electrical lighting and the constructed environment is associated with reduced exposure to sunlight during the day, increased light exposure after sunset, and a delayed timing of the circadian clock. . . . Furthermore, we find that after exposure only to natural light, the internal circadian clock synchronizes to solar time such that the beginning of the internal biological night occurs at sunset and the end of the internal biological night occurs before wake time just after sunrise." Even more interesting, the team of researchers found that levels of melatonin, the hormone that is triggered in the pineal gland in our brains to make us feel sleepy, were slower to drop in the mornings with those exposed to electric light, making them feel groggy for longer.[4]

Maybe you don't think that this is important. Perhaps, like

Thomas Edison, the coinventor of the light bulb, you think that sleep simply makes a person "unhealthy and inefficient." That the ability of the humble electric light bulb to create a whole world of fun and entertainment, of work and advancement, is worth the human cost. You wouldn't be alone: This core belief formed the basis for many of the advances of the twentieth century, in the sense that the developed world is a twenty-four-hour one, and that the stark difference between day and night is for less developed, less forward-thinking cultures. And so what if our circadian rhythms are out of whack? It's the price of progress, surely.

Well, the evidence shows that quite apart from the huge numbers of birds and mammals confused by light—one study found that as many as ten thousand birds a day die in North America by crashing into brightly lit office buildings, their compasses confused by the light source, which they mistake for the star constellations by which they navigate—the impact of electric light on our ancient systems is greater than we'd thought. A study conducted by Harvard Medical School in the early 2000s on the effects of work patterns on hospital junior doctors found that "the higher number of long shifts the doctors worked, the more likely they were to become a danger on the roadway. Interns who worked at least five long shifts a month were twice as likely to fall asleep while driving a moving vehicle, and three times more likely to fall asleep while stopped at a red light, than a colleague who worked fewer hours."[5]

But hospital doctors are the exception, right? The rest of us are just fine. Well, light pollution has been found to have a role in turning off melatonin, and if you want further evidence that artificial light interferes with our biological rhythms, you don't have to look far. A study conducted by Johanna Meijer of Leiden University Medical Center in the Netherlands showed that the mice she and her colleagues exposed to twenty-four-hour light for a period of up to six months displayed some worrying characteristics: "Studies of the animals' brain activity showed that the constant light exposure reduced the normal rhythmic patterns in the brain's central circadian pacemaker of the suprachiasmatic nuclei (SCN) by 70 per cent."[6] And crucially, this disruption resulted in a loss of muscle tone and bone density, which, notably, was reversed once the animals' normal cycle of light and dark was restored. Again, the point of this information is not to induce panic, but to show that artificial light isn't quite as benign as we'd first thought. It does have an impact on us, whether we like it or not, and the trick, as we'll discover in this book, is to use it well.

WHAT IS LIGHT?

It may seem like an obvious question: What is light? You can see it coming in your window; you can switch on an electric light in your home, or look at the moon in the sky. What difference does it make if you know what it is? But the story of light is one of trying to understand one of life's great mysteries, and if you understand something, you can truly reap its benefits. As Einstein said, "Any fool can know. The point is to understand."

Put simply, light is a form of electromagnetic radiation. But our journey to understanding this puzzled scientists for many years, with two ideas in particular competing: *Light has either been seen as a stream of extremely tiny particles with a definite color, or as a rolling sea of interacting and vibrating waves.* Why this is important is something we'll explore later. In around 300 BCE, the ancient Greek philosopher Euclid stated that the eyes possessed an inner fire and that beams of light emanated from the pupils. Euclid thought that the rays traveled outward, and that when these burning jets hit external objects, these suddenly became visible. This might seem unlikely, but many people shared Euclid's view. It was another seven hundred years before the Arab mathematician and optician Ibn al-Haytham found that light moved in straight lines, but in the opposite direction and in fact *entered into the eyes*. His empirical proof was simple yet utterly convincing. Briefly glance at the sun and notice how it feels. Burning pain? Of course. Copious amounts of light enter the eyes and strike the delicate retinas. It would seem that Ibn al-Haytham was onto something.

In 1666, the English physicist Isaac Newton prepared a darkened room and made a small hole in the window shutter. The entering sunbeam was intercepted by a triangular piece of glass he had bought at a local fun fair. (Prisms were considered playthings and toys for children at the time.) The white bundle of light was separated into a whole rainbow of brilliant colors that he projected onto the wall. Newton was religiously inclined and wanted to see the sacred seven in the spectrum: red-orange-yellow-green-blue-indigo-violet. He thought that light was made up of microscopic colored corpuscles, or cells. Green light, for example, was a bundle of tiny green particles moving very fast in linear tracks. If unimpeded, they would continue straight ahead, but if they struck a shiny surface, such as a mirror, they would be symmetrically reflected. The alleged little particles behaved much like billiard balls bouncing off a wall. Newton liked playing billiards and found this a very fitting image—and since he was a famous man, everyone agreed with him.

Newton's particle theory was taken as gospel for a very long time, until the English doctor and physicist Thomas Young conducted an inventive experiment that transformed the science of optics. A light beam was directed onto two adjacent slits on a plate. The radiation pattern from the double apertures was a huge surprise. It was not a projected image of two separate slits, but a series of alternating dark and bright fringes. They looked exactly like overlapping water waves, and no particle theory could explain this. The academic pendulum now swung swiftly to the other extreme, with the firm and dogmatic belief that light was a series of waves spreading from its source. But while this is fine, people also believed that we could see these waves, which we now know we can't.

The discoveries of William Herschel and his sister Caroline alerted us to the existence of other kinds of light beyond the visible spectrum, in this case infrared light. The German-Polish chemist and physicist Johann Ritter discovered ultraviolet light, but it was really only in the nineteenth century that discoveries in light really took shape. In 1864, the Scottish mathematician and physicist James Clerk Maxwell discovered that light is a form of electromagnetic radiation: electric and magnetic waves moving at the speed of light. The light that we can see is only one part of a much larger spectrum of electromagnetic radiation. Radio waves, microwaves, X-rays—and light—are all forms of radiation belonging to the known electromagnetic spectrum.

In 1900, the German physicist Max Planck became the father of the new quantum era. Electrical companies wanted a high output from the new and exciting invention of light bulbs, with a minimal input of energy, and asked him for the recipe. This was easier said than done, because if all the energies of light frequencies were added together, the energy demand would be infinite. Thus, Planck suggested that light only existed in discrete packets, or quanta. It took the boldness of the German-Swiss physicist Albert Einstein to bring the argument full circle, with his Nobel Prize–winning assertion, through the photoelectric effect, that light was once more a stream of particles.

So was light waves or particles? Were we back to square one again? In 1924, the French physicist Louis de Broglie settled all the arguments with a neat equation. Light was both. In the quantum world, moving objects or particles could equally well be seen as vibrations or waves. The naming was largely a matter of convenience that depended on the situation. Modern physics solves the riddle elegantly by looking at water. An undulating field of snow actually consists of many tiny snowflakes without any paradox whatsoever. The individual drops together make an ocean. And it is with this image in mind that we have arrived at our current understanding of the nature of light.

Recent developments in mixing matter and light have opened the gate to a whole new understanding of the science of optics. This makes it possible to study the process of photosynthesis and to understand it, to make new materials. Graphene is one of these, a "wonder material," which, we are told, will revolutionize everything from light bulbs to buildings to sports equipment.[7] As Andrei Seryi, director of the John Adams Institute for Accelerator Science at Oxford University, said: "It's breathtaking to think that things we thought are not connected, can in fact be converted to each other: matter and energy, particles and light. Would we be able in the future to convert energy into time and vice versa?"[8]

So we now know that light is essential, and that the balance of light and darkness is necessary for us to function as human beings; we also know that electric light has altered this balance forever. But we're hardly going to return to the cave, are we? It's unrealistic to think that we can simply turn back the clock to the time when we were hunter-gatherers, living in the dappled shade of the equatorial rain forest—although our ancient brains still respond to this type of light: Try it yourself by taking a walk in a shady park in sunlight.

We know that we are truly creatures of the modern era, with all the twenty-four-hour benefits that that entails: the great leaps and bounds in technology that help us to stay alive and to recover in the hospital, that power advances in computing and help us to better educate our children. To squander these advances would be ill-advised, not to mention impossible. However, many of us are looking at ways to mitigate the impact of the great flooding of life by electric light—from the International Dark-Sky Association to apps that mimic dusk for our phones and computers—and we are also looking at harnessing its properties for our own well-being, in therapeutic light, but also in embracing the great benefits of natural light.

Before we delve into the modern era, let's look more closely at natural light: how to make it our friend, what's good (and not so good!) for us, how we consume natural light, and how we can enjoy its benefits safely.

3

WHY DO WE NEED NATURAL LIGHT?

Light brings us the news of the Universe.

—SIR WILLIAM BRAGG

I t seems that after more than a century of enjoying the benefits of electric light, we have now come to understand that this fantastic invention cannot provide the full benefits of natural light; furthermore, our reliance on electric lighting is impacting our health in so many ways, from poor sleep and weight gain to a range of other health issues. Numerous studies have been conducted to measure the effects of natural light and, as we have seen in previous chapters, the lack of it certainly affects our sleep and our perception of the passing of time. Today, many realize there is a link between winter depression and lack of sunlight, but this was not always the case, as we learned in chapter 1 (see page 3).

But before we delve into the world of natural light, let's define what it actually is. Interestingly, seventeenth-century philosophers used "natural light" to mean things about which we humans shared basic assumptions. René Descartes was particularly keen on this definition, and on the idea that there were certain things that "could be presented to the intellect, and would leave no room for doubt."[9] The Latin term for this is the charming *lumen naturale*. How apt for a process that would "shine a light" on our human minds!

From the previous chapter we know that, scientifically, "light" is a form of electromagnetic radiation. What I mean by "natural light" is the form of electromagnetic radiation that is produced by the sun. Radio waves, microwaves, X-rays, and visible light are all forms of radiation belonging to the known electromagnetic spectrum. You don't need to worry too much about this at the moment, but it's useful to know that the spectrum's full scope and range is huge, and that we can see only a tiny part of it—the visible spectrum. Sunlight contains the full spectrum of visible light as well as the adjoining infrared and ultraviolet radiation. A simple question to start with is, Why do we need full-spectrum natural daylight? Quite simply, we cannot survive without it. Full-spectrum daylight provides body cells with vital information and activates cascades of molecular reactions.

SUNLIGHT

Direct sunshine is the finest source of light. Your entire biology is coded to it. Sunlight is environmentally friendly and absolutely free of charge. But sunlight also helps us to synthesize vitamin D, a vitamin that may have an even greater role in our health than we'd first thought. Some of us might remember the terrible disease of "rickets," in which the bones become malformed due to lack of calcium (vitamin D helps the body to absorb calcium), but researchers are currently investigating the vitamin's role in fighting off a number of other diseases, too.

*What I mean by "natural light" is
the form of electromagnetic radiation
that is produced by the sun.*

The British National Health Service, or NHS, recommends that breastfed babies and young children should take extra vitamin D, while adults who do not get out much during the summer months, such as the elderly or unwell, or those with darker skin tones, should consider a supplement throughout the year. Those who do not fall into these categories can simply take a supplement during the winter months.[10] Always consult a doctor or qualified nutritionist before taking supplements.

We can get vitamin D from our diet, by eating foods such as oily fish (salmon, mackerel), and from cod liver oil, as well as from fortified milks, egg yolks, and cheese, but recent research indicates that these dietary sources may not be as potent—a point which I'll return to in chapter 5—and there is nothing quite like a dose of daylight to boost our mood, and to tell our bodies that it's time to be awake and productive.

Interestingly, while electric light may have allowed factories to run twenty-four hours a day, natural daylight has been found to increase human productivity. One of the better-known studies in this area was undertaken in 1999 by the Heschong Mahone Group, which studied whether natural daylight had an effect on pupils' performance in schools in certain US locations. What they found was that students in a school in Fresno, California, performed 20 percent better in natural daylight.[11] Furthermore, a study conducted, somewhat ironically, by the Pacific Gas and Electric Company on daylight in a chain of stores found that checkouts located beneath a skylight reported a 40 percent increase in sales. Additionally, a later study found that "during the California power crisis of 2001, when the chain operated its stores at half-lighting power, the daylit stores had an average 5.5 percent increase in sales relative to the non-daylit stores."[12] Clearly, we humans have an inbuilt preference for natural light!

But what if you work in a gloomy office or in a location away from windows? You'll probably intuitively understand that it's not beneficial, but what you might not be aware of is the extent to which it might impact your life. In a study conducted by Northwestern University in Chicago, reported in *Psychology Today*, it was found that "compared to workers in offices without windows, those with windows in the work-place received 173 percent more white light exposure during work hours *and slept an average of 46 minutes more per night* [my italics]. Workers without windows reported lower scores than their counterparts on quality of life measures related to physical problems and vitality. They also had poorer outcomes in measures of overall sleep quality, sleep efficiency, sleep disturbances, and daytime dysfunction."[13]

The answer? If you can't change your working conditions, try to get outside: a decent dose of genuine daylight around noon is the best way to get sufficient quantities of full-spectrum light. Even an overcast day will give a surprisingly large amount of light due to the volume of the open sky. When fully fed, your skin will soon synthesize valuable vitamin D. An exposure of larger areas of skin for twenty minutes will normally suffice to fully charge the cellular reserves of this vitamin. We will look at how to do this safely on page 30.

We also need natural light to see well. The sun's rays are *parallel*. So while all artificially generated light beams originate from sources at a close distance, providing divergent rays, the enormous distance of the sun make its rays parallel. Large amounts of parallel light are close to impossible to obtain with artificial means. The sun's parallel rays enhance textural features through precise shadow play. This gives your eyes distinct information about surface detail. Also, bright sunshine will stimulate the healthy action of the retinal color cones in your eye. We'll look at this in more detail later, but like many other body tissues they need to be exercised, which means that they need strong luminous stimulation in order to function properly. But beware—sunshine can be damaging, so no staring at the sun. You can, however, gradually train your eyes to function at higher light levels, while avoiding harsh glares or reflections.

Children need to take greater care than adults, because their eyes are not fully developed; although children and adults are all exposed to the same amount of radiation, the sensitivity of children is three times higher (and many of them do not wear eye protection). Encourage your children to wear sunglasses in bright glare. However, some experts suggest that because children's pupils are a little wider than those of adults, wearing sunglasses causes the pupils to dilate, therefore letting in more sunlight. The result of this will be that your child might ultimately be more sensitive to light. Medical opinion on children wearing sunglasses varies, so, as with every parenting decision, it's wise to use common sense.

SKYLIGHT

Skylight is the second and less obvious component of daylight. It is basically diffused sunlight, and one notices it most when facing away from the sun. Skylight has a bluish hue to it and occurs when incoming sunlight is scattered in the upper stratospheric layers. Short blue wavelengths are dispersed more than any other color range, so looking up in any direction, you will get an impression of blueness. It is impossible to achieve anything similar by artificial means. Overcast skylight, on the other hand, won't help us to see detail, but provides excellent background light, which is why many artists' studios face north. When the sun is high, blue light is scattered everywhere. When the sun is low, the light has to pass through deeper layers of air, so only the long wavelengths or red/pink colors will pass through the atmospheric filter.

MOONLIGHT

You might wonder at the inclusion of moonlight here, as, technically speaking, the moon does not produce any radiation. However, moonlight is sunlight cast back by the moon, and this has an identity of its own. As we have seen, according to the laws of physics, all reflected light becomes polarized to varying degrees—that is, it moves in an orderly direction depending on the smoothness of the surface. The lunar landscape is obviously not a polished disc, so moonlight is only weakly polarized. The full moon offers very limited color vision but is certainly strong enough to show the way during nocturnal navigation. In fact, a study in *Nature* in 2003[14] discovered that the humble dung beetle used the moon's polarization to roll its ball of dung in a straight line! It has long been understood that animals can orient themselves in moonlight, and of course humans have learned to adapt to this weaker light, too. In desert cultures, strong sunlight was considered a very mixed blessing. The heat of the day would be scorching and hindered any physical work. Caravan travelers much preferred to journey in the cool of night, under a reasonably strong moon.

We know that our year is measured by Earth's journey around the sun, which takes 365 days to complete, but the four lunar phases also give us a robust time frame and form the basis of the monthly calendar. As the moon orbits the earth, it takes about 29.5 days—*moon* and *month*; see the similarity?—and different parts of it are lit up on different days, so we move from the new moon, to the "waxing," or growing, crescent moon; to a half-moon; then to "waxing gibbous," which fantastic expression simply means growing bigger, until we reach a full moon again. So the moon clearly plays an important role in the marking of time, in navigation, and also in the cycle of sea tides, even if its effects on human biology aren't as significant as we might think.

STARLIGHT

Starlight has an extremely low influx, which simply means that such low levels of light reach us that the reality is darkness. How did our early ancestors relate to natural darkness? Nightfall was probably treated with the deepest respect and even trepidation. Color vision was completely absent and all sense of spatial direction lost. Obscurity was the ultimate horror. You could not tell friend from foe, let alone discern all the nocturnal demons. Humans are not nocturnal animals. Yet despite its downsides, deep night did have some beauty and utility. The visual brain would detect where true north was; distant stars and galaxies became clearly visible as useful beacons for long-distance navigation; and stellar light would offer fixed goals during future migrations out of Africa.

So from all that we've just learned, it's clear that natural light is a "temporal marker," helping us to divide time into years and months. We also know that it is important for vitamin D synthesis and for vision. But how can we optimize the inflow of natural light in our lives? And, more important, how can we do so safely?

As we have seen, light starvation is a genuine concern for those of us who live at higher latitudes, where life during the long, dark winters can be truly troublesome. I know this to be the case from my own practice, where at the end of autumn clients will start complaining of fatigue, overeating, and low spirits in general. The effects are exacerbated if people are sun-starved after a lousy summer. The statistics bear this out: Research undertaken by Swedish academics found that young people in central Sweden reported a 20 percent incidence of SAD during the winter months, which compared with a tiny 0.1 percent in summer. (Interestingly, 26 percent of girls reported feeling affected by the winter blues, in contrast to 14 percent of boys.) When a larger group was given the same detailed questionnaire, 3 percent found that they were "severely affected" by SAD, but, tellingly, 19 percent found that their daily lives were negatively affected by the condition.[15]

Nowadays, in the developed world, 90 percent of our lives is spent indoors.

But SAD isn't just an emotional problem. Lack of sunshine poses a very real medical risk. For example, researchers undertaking a study of blood pressure in Chile discovered that those who lived farther away from the equator had higher blood pressure than those who lived closer, and while they didn't pinpoint the exact factors that influenced this, it was thought that the lack of daylight played a role.[16] Also, as we have learned, vitamin D deficiency is a very real issue for many people. But did you also know that this, too, depends on where you live? A Harvard study found that, except during the summer months, our skin will make very little—if any—vitamin D if we live either 37 degrees above or below the equator.[17] Also, blind people and cataract patients have reduced light inputs and consequently lower levels of vital body hormones.

You may be thinking, *Where I live, the sun is always shining—I don't have a problem.* Well, think again. The most widespread form of daylight starvation stems from our relatively recent retreat to indoor life. Nowadays, in the developed world, 90 percent of our lives is spent indoors. Shutters, curtains, and dark sunglasses may additionally cut out any remaining daylight. Computer screens are switched on all day, but natural light is largely limited.

NAVIGATING WITHOUT THE SUN

We know that insects have excellent navigation skills, and so did our ancestors, the Vikings. They navigated the waters between their native Norway and North America, Scotland, and Ireland without a compass, and on bright days they would have used the sun to do so. However, quite how they did so on days when they couldn't see the sun used to be something of a mystery. It was suggested by the Danish archaeologist Thorhild Ramskou that they may have used what they called *sunstone*, a chunk of clear crystal called an *Icelandic spar*, but how wasn't entirely clear, particularly when the sun wasn't visible—which it quite frequently would not have been in the gloomy North Atlantic. The answer lies in polarization, or the direction in which light vibrates.

The physicist Guy Ropars from the University of Rennes, in France, conducted an experiment with a piece of Icelandic spar, which had been found on a shipwreck off the Channel Island of Alderney. According to *National Geographic* magazine, researchers hit the crystal with a beam of partly polarized light and rotated the crystal until they found the spot where the two beams met. It is thought that the Vikings may have marked this spot for use on cloudy days. Then the researchers sent volunteers outside on a cloudy day to see if they could use the sunstone to locate the sun's position—which they could do to a remarkable degree of accuracy. They found that "by rotating the crystal against the human eye until the darkness of the two shadows were equal, the sun's position can be pinpointed with remarkable accuracy."[18]

GOOD SUN SENSE

Many of us have fully taken on board the need to protect ourselves from the sun's harmful rays. It is true that excessive exposure to the sun's ultraviolet rays UVA and UVB can cause you to burn. We also know that repeated exposure to the sun can be a cause of skin cancer and can age the skin prematurely. However, rather than shunning the sun completely, we need to embrace its benefits wisely.

Some professionals tell us that we can spend up to twenty minutes in the sun before our skin will begin to burn. However, this depends on the strength of the UV rays, which vary according to the weather and time of year, and also your skin type. For example, you might not be aware that spring sunshine—lovely as it is—has strong UV rays, so you may well burn, even though it doesn't yet feel "hot."[19] If you have a paler or freckled complexion, you will burn more quickly, but if your skin is darker, you will burn more slowly—but you will still burn! The key is to take precautions so that you can enjoy outdoor life without compromising on safety. So limit your exposure during the hottest time of the day, between 10 a.m. and 4 p.m. in the summertime, and check the UV index for your city or country, which will tell you how powerful the UV rays are on a particular day or time (many weather-forecasting organizations will include this on their websites, and the World Health Organization [WHO] has a listing of world cities and the average UV index in each during the twelve months of the year). And when exposing your skin to sunlight, try not to overdo your face and hands, which will generally see a little too much of the sun; concentrate on exposing larger areas of skin for short periods. For more on this, see page 68.

Also, research your sunscreen carefully. Note that the higher the SPF, the smaller the difference in UV protection: For example, a sunscreen with an SPF of 30 will filter out around 97 percent of UVB rays, but an SPF of 50 will only filter out an extra 1 percent at 98 percent. The higher the SPF, the smaller the difference. Look out for words like *broad spectrum*, which mean the sunscreen will filter out UVA and UVB rays. Also check just how "waterproof" your sunscreen is—don't leave it to chance, but reapply after you've been for your swim; this applies particularly to children, who are in and out of the water all the time. The same goes for "sweat-proof" creams.

So the lesson is, spend more time outdoors, but be safe. There's nothing like a walk at lunchtime to perk you up and to give you your daily dose of vitamin D, as well as to make you

happier and more productive, but there's no need to lie under a
hot sun or to sacrifice your skin to it to gain the psychological
and physical benefits.

A few simple actions will improve your—*safe*—exposure to
sunlight:

Open the shutters

Don't spend your life in constant obscurity behind sealed shutters, curtains, and blinds. Let some natural light into your home.
Dappled light is very pleasant and allows selected portions of
sun rays to enter. A healthy dose of sunlight, taken with care,
is especially important if you have a dark complexion, as weak
light cannot penetrate your protective skin deeply enough to
feed the blood in the underlying capillaries. Also, while your
skin contains large amounts of the brown pigment melanin, this
very thing will make it harder for you to absorb vitamin D.

Avoid gloomy interiors

It may seem unrealistic to those of us who live in basement
apartments or who work in windowless offices, but if at all possible, avoid these gloomy environments. They affect your mood
and, as we've seen, they also affect your well-being. Even fancy
modern shopping plazas or offices with shaded windows present
problems, particularly if you plan to stay all day in them. Dark
interiors are not suitable for healthy light consumers, because
you'll be constantly starved of good daylight, which will upset
your biological rhythms and could even eventually shorten your
life span. For evidence of this, we need look no further than
that uniquely twentieth- and twenty-first-century invention:
shift work. With as many as 20 percent of us working shifts,

this is certainly part of modern life now, but there have been a number of studies that have shown shift workers are at higher risk of certain serious conditions. Additionally, many shift workers performed more poorly on cognitive tests and, according to *Medical News Today*, in 2007 the WHO decided to classify night-shift work as a potential carcinogen, due to the disruption of the body's circadian rhythms.[20]

Ditch the black

We have often been told that wearing black in heat is a no-no. In fact, in an interesting little experiment titled "Why Do Bedouins Wear Black Robes in Hot Deserts?" four scientists pondered the conundrum of how the Bedouin people, who, after all, had lived in deserts for thousands of years, frequently wore black robes without any difficulty. They found, by placing an unfortunate volunteer in a variety of garments in the baking desert heat, that while black robes did conduct more heat, the heat was lost before it hit the skin, because the looseness of the clothing made the heat flow off the body.[21] However, this amusing anecdote conceals a more serious issue: that wearing dark barriers to sunlight on the *head* can affect how sunlight is absorbed in the body. According to the International Osteoporosis Foundation, "hypovitaminosis D"—in other words, a lack of this essential vitamin—is a real issue in Middle Eastern countries. Any barriers to sunlight—such as veils, dark hats, hoods, or scarves covering the head—may affect future bone health.[22]

Use sunglasses wisely

When it comes to sunglasses, again, less is most definitely more: Wearing sunglasses in, say, the living room or deep shade is inadvisable, as your eyes will not be able to send the correct messages to your poor brain! However, of course it's sensible to wear them to reduce glare when sailing or skiing—nobody wants a case of snow blindness, which, while temporary, is painful. However, some eye problems, like macular degeneration or cataracts, are thought to be *in part* due to high levels of sun exposure, so it seems sensible to protect our eyes, but not to completely avoid natural light.

WHAT SHOULD YOU LOOK OUT FOR WHEN YOU ARE BUYING SUNGLASSES?

- Expensive is not necessarily best. In a range of tests conducted for a British daily newspaper, an optometrist rated a 99p pair of sunglasses 10/10 in terms of UV protection. Of course, I'm not recommending that you go out and buy the cheapest pair you can find. *What you do need to be sure about is that the label on the glasses says either "CE" or "UV400."* Note that standards in Europe are not quite as rigorous as they are in, say, Australia. If in doubt, feel free to take your sunglasses into an optician to test the UV filter quality.

- The color of the tint on the sunglasses makes no difference in regard to the UV protection. Just because the lens is dark doesn't mean that the glasses will filter out more harmful rays.

- Make sure that the frames cover your whole eye, with no gaps for light to get in.

- When it comes to children, exercise caution when buying sunglasses. It's a good idea to encourage children to wear sunglasses when they will be in the sun for long periods of time, or while playing sports in bright sunshine, but many medical experts suggest that children do not need to wear sunglasses at all times. Let common sense be your guide.

Go easy on skin art

Tattoos contain metallic salts in the form of oxides and sulphides, along with organic dyes or plastics. Many of these colored chemicals were originally intended for use in printer inks and automobile paints. Phototoxic reactions from exposure to sunlight have been reported, but long-term effects of interaction with strong light are largely unknown. As a rule of thumb, the larger the area covered by a tattoo, the higher the risk. Likewise, daily use of heavy makeup can be harmful, partly because of its chemical content and partly because it can act as a sunscreen, if, indeed, it contains an SPF—heavy sunscreens starve us of the positive effects of sunlight.

So there we have it: Natural light is to be embraced for its life-enhancing qualities, and for the incredible way it helps our bodies to function. We all need a little light in our lives to improve our mood and productivity, but we also need to respect the power of the sun and take sensible precautions to keep ourselves healthy and happy.

ELECTRIC LIGHT

I find out what the world needs.
Then, I go ahead and invent it.

—THOMAS EDISON

Any discussion of electric light wouldn't be possible without the man who said the above. The American inventor Thomas Edison was responsible for so many amazing things, from the earliest record player—the phonograph—to the Dictaphone, and even an early movie camera. He also took out an enormous 2,332 patents in his lifetime of work. However, his most remarkable invention is that of the light bulb, which he shared with the Englishman Joseph Swan. In his famous Menlo Park, New Jersey, lab, Edison oversaw an industrial process of invention that was to change the course of the twentieth century.

Before Edison and Swan's light-bulb moment, energy was produced by smelly, dirty gas and coal. Following the production of the very first incandescent electric light bulb in 1879,

Edison declared, "We will make electricity so cheap that only the rich will burn candles." Edison was true to his word, setting up his own electricity company, the Edison Electric Light Company. The rest is history, as they say, but the power of this energy—which wasn't clean at first, incidentally, as coal was needed to fire generators—was used in the creation of the world we know today, of brightly lit theaters and cinemas, factories that run day and night, and a domestic life that runs more smoothly thanks to refrigerators, air conditioners, dishwashers, and washing machines. Where would we be without electricity?

When electric light became widespread, it was seen as a boon, a sign that the world was entering a new era. However, what we now know is that electricity, while an essential part of our lives, isn't as straightforward as it first seemed. We are becoming increasingly aware of the unintended consequences of our love affair with electric light, from light pollution to the fatigue, insomnia, and disrupted body rhythms that come with overconsumption. Our twenty-four-hour world impacts much more than we'd thought on our ancient selves.

However, as with so many things, the trick is to increase our knowledge of this energy source and our awareness of it, so that we can use it sensibly. Before we learn more about the different kinds of electric light and how they affect us, let's learn a little bit more about the basics.

ELECTRIC LIGHTING FOR THE HOME

When you are looking at buying electric bulbs and lamps for the home, you might notice the words *lux* and *lumens*. These are measurements of light intensity, with one lux roughly comparing to the illumination provided by a full moon. In nature, sunlight ranges from 32,000 to 100,000 lux, so very bright! By comparison, on a clear day, ambient outdoor light is about 400 lux, and on a gloomy day it can measure just 100 lux.

When lighting a space, we consider lumens. A lumen is a standardized unit of measurement for the total amount of light produced by a light source, such as a lamp. One lux is defined as being equivalent to one lumen spread over an area of one square meter.

How much light do we need for various activities? Some current standard recommendations are: 100 lux in a living room, 500 lux in an office, and 1,000 lux for precision work. Of course, this will depend on the size of the room and what kind of light you will be using (for more about lux, lumens, and room lights, see page 109). The European Union recommends 500 lux as adequate illumination for an office desk. This is considered a good and stimulating light level for intellectual efforts. But is it really? As we have seen, many office workers are tired at the end of the day. Consider the contrast of a sunny Florida beach: Shimmering sunlight backed by reflecting white sands and glittering waters will easily provide an impressive 100,000 lux. But is this extreme dose an obvious overload? No. This enormous level of light automatically boosts our neuronal batteries. It makes us feel buoyant and happy, as it corresponds to the luminosity of our biological roots near the equator.

The European Union recommends 500 lux as adequate illumination for an office desk. This is considered a good and stimulating light level for intellectual efforts. But is it really?

Let's look at another couple of terms that might be helpful. The first of these is *color temperature*. Simply put, it means the relationship between the color of light and the temperature of its source. Let's look at the Kelvin color temperature scale. This measures the temperature of light, and the way it does so is by imagining what scientists call a "black body" object—such as a lamp filament—being heated. At some point, this lamp filament will get hotter and begin to glow. As it gets hotter, the color shifts from deep red, to orange, to yellow, and then on to bluish white. In light sources such as this, we call them "incandescent radiators," and they allow us to see the full color spectrum (see page 44).[23] While direct daylight (white light) corresponds to a color temperature of around 6,000K, the ambient background of the blue sky can reach a temperature of 20,000K. This might seem like Greek to you, but where it becomes more relevant is when it comes to artificial light. Many companies claim that their products mimic the full spectrum of natural daylight, but is this true? The answer lies in color temperature!

We know that plants can grow under artificial lights that imitate the sun, because we see the results when we buy a bunch of tulips in December. Even more remarkably, lights have been developed that will mimic the conditions that particular plants need for growth. This technology has actually been around for a long time, since its discovery by a Russian botanist named Andrei Famintsyn—but how are humans affected by the so-called full-spectrum light in these lights?

To ascertain this, we need to consider the color temperature, but also to look at the color rendering index (CRI). What this does is measure the accuracy of either real or perceived colors when a light is compared with a natural light.

The Color Rendering Index (CRI)

The CRI measures values from 0 to 100, with 100 indicating that colors are most accurately represented when viewed under an artificial light source. As you can imagine, this is very important to photographers, art restorers, and historians, but it's also important for the rest of us. It can have an impact when we are examining manufacturers' claims for their "daylight" or "full-spectrum" lighting products. For example, the orange glow of a streetlamp has a "negative" CRI, meaning that you won't be able to see color clearly; try standing under a streetlight and looking at your clothes to see how it distorts their color. A fluorescent light will give you a CRI of about 80 (out of a possible 100), and an LED will bring you closer to 90.

Light with a high color rendering will provide correct information to the visual brain, and the emotional impression will be one of beauty. The cognitive impression will be one of precision and exactness, like the experience of listening to a well-tuned instrument.

Of course, household electricity can never generate the raw photonic power of the sun. As a result, our indoor environments are often lacking in sufficient light. Without adequate lighting for the tasks we want to perform, our eyes will suffer and our brains will protest. Creating an optimal lighting plan involves many different factors, as we will discover. But the single most important thing you can do to improve your electric light diet is to choose *efficient* light bulbs emitting *quality* light. What do we mean by this?

THE EFFICIENCY OF LIGHT BULBS

The luminous output of a light source is measured in lumens. The energy needed to generate this output is measured in watts. The efficiency of a light bulb is therefore indicated as lumens per watt (lm/W). This means the amount of light that is produced by a certain number of watts, i.e., electrical power. The table opposite gives you an idea of the efficiency of different light sources; the values are only examples and may vary between different brands, especially when it comes to LEDs, for which no international standards exist. For your information, OLED means "organic light-emitting diode," and I'll explain what this means below.

Standard incandescent	10–15 lm/W
Halogen incandescent	15–30 lm/W
Fluorescent tube	50–100 lm/W
OLED	70–100 lm/W
LED	100–150 lm/W

As you can see, the standard incandescent light bulb does not produce a lot of light for the amount of energy it uses, in contrast to the LED, which produces a lot more light. Choosing efficient light bulbs makes good environmental sense, because these bulbs will give you a lot more light for your electricity usage and will lower your electricity bill. Indeed, there has been something of a race recently to produce the first 200-lumens-per-watt light bulb, so you can imagine the energy savings.

Study the technical specifications presented by different lamp manufacturers—the fine print that nobody usually bothers to read. Detailed data and guidance on each type of light source can be found below. But remember, buy the best-quality lighting that you can afford, and don't be afraid to ask questions of your lighting supplier. You are the customer, and you are in the driver's seat. Most hardware stores will have someone knowledgeable to advise you, but if you are purchasing in a supermarket or even online, do your research first to make sure you know what you are buying.

Everyday lighting

Standard incandescent is the traditional light bulb most of us recognize, containing thin strands of glowing tungsten. These old standard bulbs function much better as radiators of heat than as light sources, as most of their emission lies in the infrared range, with 97 percent heat and only 3 percent visible light. This humble bulb may have lit many a dingy student apartment, but the waste of energy involved is not acceptable in our environmentally conscious world. This bulb was banned in Europe in 2009 and globally in 2014. New ones should not have been produced after that date.

A standard incandescent bulb has a short life span of typically 1,000 hours. It gives a full output of light during its whole life cycle, but then the fine wire suddenly snaps and the whole thing goes dark. Dimming is simply achieved by reducing the current. Cheap to produce and involving few toxic elements, the bulb is also easy to recycle. It has a distinct orange glow, which is cosmetically charming but also sleep-inducing.

Halogen incandescent light is generated by an incandescent lamp of a similar construction to the standard bulb, but the tungsten filament is surrounded by reactive and protective halogen gases. The fine thread can be heated to higher temperatures, and some of the metal atoms will evaporate into the surrounding gas. The gaseous metals combine chemically with the halogens and redeposit on the heated wire. The metal recycles itself over and over until the slender tungsten filament eventually breaks. The process is more efficient than that of a standard bulb, as the elevated temperature generates more quality light and less thermal waste.

Quality halogen lamps normally have a lifetime of 4,000 hours and provide light fully during their life cycle before abruptly going dark. This makes them more expensive than traditional incandescent bulbs, but the energy conversion is better. Halogens involve more electronics, and the bulbs are made of quartz, which is not environmentally friendly to recycle. They still generate a lot of waste heat, and it is possible they may be withdrawn from the market in the future.

A halogen bulb is described as a "thermal radiator," which, as we'll remember from our explanation earlier, means that it makes colors "true." Its spectrum contains more blue and violet than the standard lamp and appears more neutrally white, which is why halogen lights are well suited to the display of attractive goods and visually demanding precision work. They are fed by direct current that never pulsates or flickers. Halogen incandescent is the best solar imitation commercially available, and your brain simply loves it. It may not be the most efficient, but from a human perspective it is the healthiest electric source for everyday use.

The European Union first wanted to ban *all* incandescent bulbs, but modern halogens have been modified and now it seems they will stay for the time being.

Standard fluorescent light is produced through a completely different technology. It is generated by a gaseous mixture of rarefied mercury with argon sealed off in a long glass tube internally coated with phosphors. Older fluorescent tubes were fitted with low-frequency drivers that generated very annoying pulsations, but modern ones must by law have higher frequencies. Nonetheless, even though these ultra-quick pulsations are in theory invisible to the human eye, mechanically flashing light is known to be irritating to the nerves and brain. Fluorescent light is not good for your sensitive biological system.

As those of us who work under fluorescent lights know, they are not ideal for color rendering either. Dimming is also difficult and requires special fixtures, but the tubes do have advantages: They are cheap to buy and have extremely high energy conversion, plus a long life span of up to 10,000 burning hours, which makes them a popular choice for offices. Light tubes will not abruptly go dark but will slowly dim and start to pulsate when the aging electrodes corrode.

One area where care is needed is in the recycling process. Fluorescent lights contain electronics, phosphor, and, worst of all, mercury. Particularly in gaseous form and in nanoscale dilutions, mercury is a lethal poison. You will need to take great care in removing mercury tube lights, particularly around children. Better still, avoid using fluorescent tubes in the home—there are other, better alternatives.

Compact fluorescent lights (CFLs) are small fluorescent tubes that you'll see in a spiral pattern or in a double loop in some fittings, and they will often fit into incandescent bulb sockets. Sometimes you'll see these referred to as "energy saving" lights. All well and good, and yes, they do last a lot longer than their predecessors, the humble incandescent, but . . . the tubes can have cracks in the coating where hard ultraviolet rays can escape, and any UV isn't good for you. Additionally, they are hard to recycle, needing to be disposed of by recycling centers that cater to this type of bulb, and they contain mercury in their fragile glass coils, which is not safe. Many people now favor LED lights.

LEDs may seem like a modern invention, but they've been around for a long time. Originally, when they first appeared in the 1960s, they were used in such things as digital clocks and as indicator lights on circuit boards. Their inventor, Nick Holonyak, was actually trying to create a laser in his job as a scientist at General Electric, but he was beaten to it, and the result of his efforts was a semiconductor light, which was red in color. Interestingly, it took a long time for LEDs to become a commonplace item, even though this sophisticated technology may well be the standard light source of the future.

The way LEDs are made is that compact layers of semiconducting diodes are sandwiched together. LEDs can therefore be made minutely small, and a square millimeter will suffice for an ordinary reading lamp. They are also really easy to dim and focus. Current LED models have considerable lifetimes: 50,000 hours is realistic, and future models are estimated to double that figure, which will interest those who want to place them in inaccessible places like very high ceilings. LEDs are, in principle, maintenance-free.

So far, so good, but the manufacture of LEDs involves rare and toxic minerals, including arsenic and lead. Researchers at the University of California conducted experiments on red LEDs and found that they contained substantially more lead than permissible, as well as high levels of nickel and copper. While these might not be harmful on a small scale, the researchers urged consumers to be cautious when disposing of LEDs.[24]

Current LED models have considerable lifetimes:
50,000 hours is realistic, and future models
are estimated to double that figure, which
will interest those who want to place them in
inaccessible places like very high ceilings.

They are tiny in size and consume a minimum of electricity, yet LED output is very, very bright. A study led by the German scientist Christopher Kyba found that, according to *Science Advances*, "the amount of artificial light coming from Earth's surface at night has increased in radiance and extent by 2 percent every year for the past four years, driven by the rapid adoption of bright LEDs and development."[25] Furthermore, a UK study found that artificial light may be making biological spring come sooner, with trees coming into bud a week earlier than normal.[26] It is thought that the phenomenon is partly caused by the lights themselves, which trick trees into thinking that spring is happening earlier, but also by the heat the lights emit into the air.

OLED is an acronym for "organic light-emitting diode," and you may have seen the name on some new—and expensive!— TV sets. OLEDs are thin layers of organic plastics sandwiched between two conducting plates, which radiate white light when exposed to the electric current. OLEDs are considered to produce an excellent picture quality, but as yet are not produced in high enough numbers to be attainable for the average TV viewer.

You will also possibly be aware of the other common usage for OLEDs: computer and mobile phone displays, as well as digital cameras. OLEDs refresh so much faster than LEDs that any device can bring up the information you want with incredible speed. Also, because of their flexibility, OLEDs make large displays possible, and may well be used in the billboards of the future. However, OLEDs do have their limitations: They are as yet prohibitively expensive, and because their emitted light radiates in all directions, they can't be used in focused tasks like sewing or soldering.

Filament LED lamps look almost exactly like antique incandescent bulbs with large decorative filaments. They are composed of miniature LEDs mounted on transparent support threads and are intended to mimic the incandescent bulb. The light from a filament LED is uniform and even, and another benefit is that they are highly efficient—but if you are looking for "true" color rendering, you won't find their orange light appealing.

Other light sources

Neon—this "noble gas" has really captured the imagination, from its discovery by William Ramsay in 1898, to the brightly lit Times Square, which was the creation of the 1930s advertising executive Douglas Leigh, who endowed his creations with special effects, such as smoke, floating bubbles, and steaming coffeepots. Leigh also lit up the Empire State Building, and his Bond Clothing sign, complete with sixty-six-foot-high figures and a giant waterfall, was a wonder of the 1940s and symbolized the growing power of America in the twentieth century. Indeed, according to the *New York Times*, when blackouts occurred during the war years, Leigh wasn't deterred, creating a huge advertisement for Camel cigarettes instead, which blew out rings of smoke.[27]

The way neon light is created is that it is trapped in a clear glass tube, to which electricity is applied, but did you know that applying electricity to neon gas will give you only the color orange? Different gases are used to create different colors. Helium will produce yellow, and hydrogen red, for example.

Digital projectors are another light source. They are made to operate in daylight and therefore have a very high luminous efficiency. They incorporate powerful lamps with a sharp bluish light that makes all colors look washed-out. Many use mercury vapor as a luminous medium, and their irregular spectral spikes put a definite strain on your eyes.

Xenon bulbs provide the finest sunshine copy available. Their main use is in commercial cinemas for quality projectors where accuracy really counts. The technology of the xenon bulb is complicated, but the noble gas xenon is ignited under high pressure, and temperatures between the electrodes reach solar levels.

Metal halide lamps are often used in industrial settings and in sports grounds or airports, because they generate enormous amounts of bright white light. Because they are relatively energy-efficient, they are a popular choice for public areas, but that lovely bright light comes at the considerable cost of light pollution.

Alternative light sources

Before we leave the world of lighting, let's consider two other forms, which, while not electric, may still play a part in our lives. Firstly, candles, which we love because they flatter our complexions and are soothing and pretty. Go easy on them. Used sparingly, they are fine, but a large quantity of candles will consume the oxygen in a room and could leave you with a nasty headache, as our ancestors found: Candles were once used to light concert halls, and many in the audience would find themselves listening to their favorite piece of music with growing pain in their heads. Furthermore, candles produce carbon dioxide and carbon monoxide, dangerous gases that are also odorless. Again, using a small number of candles in a well-ventilated room won't be a problem, but it pays to be candle-aware. And always put your candle out when you are going to bed—they are a fire hazard.

For many people in the developing world, kerosene lamps still fill a gap as a functional light source. They flicker less than candles and have a higher output, but their heavy orange cast makes them almost as bad for reading.

GOOD-QUALITY LIGHTING

So now that you know about lighting in technical terms, what about good-quality lighting? Determining what exactly that is among the plethora of marketing claims of lights as "daylight equivalent" or "natural spectrum" can be a tricky business. *True*, *pure*, and *ergonomic* are all terms you may have come across. These all certainly sound natural and beneficial, but often their uneven spectra and poor color rendering will give you visual indigestion. If you have a tendency to suffer from migraines, vertigo, or chronic fatigue, you should avoid fluorescent lighting. The electronic flicker even in more modern versions aggravates rapid and chaotic eye movements known as *nystagmus*.

If you are lucky enough to be building your own home, this gives you an excellent chance to get exactly the lighting you want, but be prepared to spend that little bit extra to get it right. You might be surprised to hear that many lighting designers recommend spending as much on lighting as on windows, but think about it—for much of the population, the indoors, where they are surrounded by artificial light, will be their environment for 90 percent of the time, so it pays to get it right. If you plan ahead, you'll be able to get the light that you want in the places that you want. Newer lighting systems can be controlled from one central "button" or from a tablet, but, as many lighting designers will tell you, LED fittings are flexible but a bit more complex than our old friend the incandescent bulb. Don't be afraid to ask questions, or to consult one of the many technical lighting guides available online or at your home store. We'll be discussing lighting in the home in chapter 7 (see page 101), but the key thing is to plan.

LEARNING TO BE SCREEN-SAVVY

In the midst of our technological revolution, it can be hard to look at the issue of screens and light objectively. We are so attached to the wonders of our smartphones and tablet devices! But when you think about it, you rarely look straight into a light source for any length of time, yet you will look at your screen sometimes for hours at a time. Quite naturally, this will take a toll on your eyes.

We just looked at LEDs, and LED screens are part of our lives in so many ways. Compact sources such as computer displays, laptops, tablets, and mobile phones all use them. They are meant to imitate full-spectrum light with a high level of blue. This is the optic signature of daylight, as we know, but we also know that we often work at monitor screens late in the evening. All wrong from our ancient biological perspective, but necessary for so many of us in our twenty-four-hour world.

Blue light

It's important for us to know just what effect this late-night blue light is having on us. Put simply, blue light affects production of melatonin—the sleep hormone. We know this thanks to a study conducted by Shigekazu Higuchi and his team at the Akita University School of Medicine in Japan, which tested the effects of blue light on healthy young males and found that, among other things, the brightness of the computer screen affected the user's melatonin levels, but also raised his body temperature.[28] This is significant, because our body temperature drops when we are getting ready for sleep. And since this study was conducted over fifteen years ago, computer screens have gotten brighter!

And not only do computers affect our sleep, they also affect our eyes. Think about it: all that focusing and refocusing, looking at flickering pictures, all that glare. And your poor eyes have to constantly tell your brain what to do. Doctors call the range of eye problems caused by computers "computer vision syndrome," and, worryingly, they estimate that as many as 50 to 80 percent of us might suffer from it. However, there are very simple things that you can do to minimize problems:

COMPUTER CARE

- Follow the 20-20-20 rule. Look away from your screen every 20 minutes, for 20 seconds, at an object 20 feet away to give your eyes a break.
- Blink more often. Many of us stare at a screen without realizing we forget to blink, making our eyes drier.

- Fit your computer with an anti-glare monitor, or use your settings to change the background to that shade of forest green that so nicely replicates our ancient life in dappled shade. At evening time, go for orange, that restful glow that will make us feel sleepy. There are many "orange" filters, such as f.lux, available online.

- Make sure your computer is the correct distance away from you. No sticking your face up close to it! As a rule of thumb, it should be 20 to 40 inches from your eyes. If you find you can't see at that distance, simply make the text size bigger.

- Use the nighttime setting on your mobile phone.

- Parents, be aware of the impact of blue light on your children's delicate retinas. Blue LEDs might have won their Japanese inventors a Nobel Prize, but they can be harsh. It is wise to get your children to take regular breaks from the screen, and not to expose them to screens at a very young age.

Take blue light seriously: according to Dr. Ronald Melton in the *Review of Optometry*, blue light reaches deeper into the eye and is more likely to affect the back of the eye. Blue light is emitted by the sun, so it has always been around, but newer forms of lighting and our reliance on devices have increased the threat. Melton tells us that the CFLs we discussed on page 45 contain about 25 percent blue light, and LEDs 35 percent.[29] And, as LEDs will probably comprise the vast majority of our lighting in the near future, it's clear that we need to mind our eyesight and guard against macular degeneration. The fovea centralis is a small area of tightly packed cones located near the center of the retina and is responsible for what we see straight in front of us. It is covered by a yellow protective protein layer, the macula lutea. If the macula is damaged or degenerates, as in old age, central vision, and especially color vision, will be impaired.

The optical world is catching on to this and many companies now produce "blue-blocking" lenses, which are particularly helpful to patients at risk of blue-light damage.

Screen flicker

We also have to be aware of the problem of screen flicker. The dimming of computer screens is only virtual, and done via so-called pulse modulation. This means that while the light level stays bright, it's chopped up into small pulses to give you the illusion that the screen is darkening. You won't notice it, because it all happens far too fast for the brain to detect, but your nervous system will still react to it.

HOW TO REDUCE YOUR EXPOSURE TO SCREEN FLICKER

- Set the light on your computer to a constant maximum to get rid of the flicker pulse. Avoid dimming the screen electronically, but instead use orange-toned sunglasses while using the computer. You might think that you look foolish in orange sunglasses, but looking a bit silly is a small price to pay for your eye health. Many outlets also now sell "blue-light-blocking eyewear."

- If you'll be reading a large amount of text, such as a report or even a book, print it out. Paper is so much more restful on the eye, and your brain will absorb the information more easily. The issue is a conflicting one because of the impact on the environment, so do be mindful with your printing.

- Avoid watching movies on a TV or tablet if you possibly can, and settle for shorter shows if possible. Try not to binge-watch! Opt for the cinema if you must catch the latest *Star Wars*—it's better for your eyes. More important, if you want your children to have a good night's sleep, avoid putting them in front of a flickering screen after supper. Encourage them to think that the time before bedtime is for reading a good book.

WHO'S AFRAID OF THE DARK?

After all the discussion on the benefits and hazards of electric light, now seems a good time to look at darkness. When was the last time many of us encountered a truly dark night? Or were able to see the Milky Way in the night sky? Perhaps you don't think this is important, but quite apart from the aesthetics, light pollution affects us in a number of other—unhealthy— ways. For a start, if our goal is to reduce energy consumption, excess lighting certainly won't help, nor will it help the many animals with whom we share the planet. Anyone who has seen footage of sea turtles making their way onto a Florida highway to nest, disoriented by the lights and being run over by motorists, will understand the impact of our love of electric light on animals. Furthermore, nocturnal animals no longer receive their nighttime cues to hunt, or for their prey to hide; insect populations, drawn to artificial lights, are becoming depleted; and, as we read in chapter 2, birds are becoming confused by bright city lights, their inner compasses no longer leading them in the right direction.

The International Dark-Sky Association has interesting data on the dangers of light pollution, and one of their notable discoveries is that brighter lights do not necessarily deter crime. They cite a number of studies that found that street lighting had no visible impact on crime, or indeed seemed to draw crime to them. A study in the *Journal of Epidemiology & Community Health* found "little evidence of the harmful effects of switch-off, part-night lighting, dimming . . . on road collisions or crime in England and Wales."[30] This is a controversial point of view, and many, including women, will find brightly lit areas safer for walking alone at night, but the findings do show that we might not need as much light as we thought. Perhaps the key is, light where it is needed, but not the clashing cacophony of light sources that have become part of modern life.

If you'd like to see just how brightly lit your area or country is, you can look at the world atlas of artificial night sky brightness, which shows us that 80 percent of the world's population lives with the "skyglow" of artificial light. In Europe and America, that climbs to a scary 99 percent. NASA's Blue Marble Navigator will also provide you with clear pictures of your country's light-pollution problem.

So what can we do to reduce our contribution to global light pollution? Well, for a start, we can adjust outdoor lights so that their light shines down, not up, and only reaches specific areas, so they don't fill the whole neighborhood with a glow. Also, according to the Dark-Sky Association we need to fit our lights with motion sensors and dimmer switches, so that the least light possible is used, and we should install lighting only where needed. Inside the home, the same applies: Don't use brighter lights than necessary, and encourage your children to learn to sleep with the lights off, or with the dimmest light possible.

Using heavy, tight-fitting curtains or blackout blinds in the bedroom is a good start in blocking unwanted rays, but don't forget those pesky electronic devices. Carefully mask all luminous monitors and signal diodes, or, better still, switch them off.

One of the most enjoyable ways to return to black, velvety night is to go back to nature. Camping at night will really train your eyes to see better in the dark, as well as allow you to enjoy the night sky. And better still, if you spend a whole weekend in nature, your body clock will quickly get the hang of darkness versus light, which is so much better for your health.

5

SUPER LIGHTS

Where the sun cannot enter, the doctor
must come instead.

—OLD ITALIAN PROVERB

We have now looked closely at both natural and artificial light, but there is another group of lights that I like to call "super lights," because of their great benefits to humans. To understand their power, let's go back to our old friend Norman Rosenthal, who correctly diagnosed the problem of seasonal affective disorder (SAD). Reduced levels of sunlight, particularly for those of us who live some distance from the equator, can disrupt the biological clock, and can also cause our serotonin levels to drop. And as serotonin is known to affect mood, this can cause problems for some of us.

THE POWER OF WHITE LIGHT

When Dr. Rosenthal and his team first discovered SAD, the answer to this light depletion was thought to be . . . well, light! But of a specific kind, which was then called *white light*. White light is simply the sum of all the visible light in the spectrum, and Dr. Rosenthal tried to replicate it using fluorescent tubes. He was essentially right: Artificial light can indeed fool the brain into summer mode, but as electric light is far weaker than the sun, very long sessions were needed to stimulate the pineal gland (known as the "third eye," which produces melatonin) into action. When Dr. Rosenthal began his work with patients, two hours a day for two weeks was the standard treatment—too slow for patients and practitioners. Since that time, many discoveries have been made that have helped to refine the process, such as that by two researchers at the New York State Psychiatric Institute, Professor Michael Terman and Jiuan Su Terman, who discovered that light therapy of 10,000 lux was most beneficial for SAD sufferers.

Now, light boxes and dawn simulators are freely available, as are therapeutic desk lamps and even glasses.[31] Bigger white boxes are certainly better, but avoid fluorescent tubes, as they contain mercury. I prefer colored monochromatic light to white light, as this works faster. Additionally, the SAD organization in the UK[32] has further tips to help you decide what you need:

- ‣ Make sure your SAD light box is "medically certified"—that is, certified by an organization known as MHRA. That's the Medicines and Healthcare Products Regulatory Agency in the United Kingdom.

- ‣ Make sure that it is of sufficient lux to actually make a difference: 2,500 lux is the minimum, but you might need to spend longer with it to benefit; 10,000 lux is considered to be most beneficial, and your treatment time will be around 15 to 20 minutes every morning, sometimes longer. As a rule of thumb, the stronger the light, the shorter the treatment, but the greater the expense—so if you have a busy lifestyle, you might well have to pay more.

- Bulb tube or LED? Cost may be an issue here, as LEDs last longer and you won't have to replace the bulb tube as often. However, according to Dr. Rosenthal, bulb tubes are more effective, as LEDs haven't been tested as much, so do your research!

- Use your light box earlier in the day—otherwise it could keep you awake.

- Newer research favors blue light as opposed to white, due in part to shorter treatment times, but as SADA.org.uk has pointed out, blue light is not suitable for those with eye conditions, or those who suffer from migraines. If in doubt, check with your GP or with an expert in the SAD field.

- Try before you buy. Many SAD light-box suppliers will allow a trial period for you to test the box—avail of this to make sure that this expensive purchase is absolutely right for you. Many people find light therapy helpful with SAD, but others find a course of cognitive behavioral therapy useful. Talk to your GP about what's right for you.

CASE STUDY:
USING A LIGHT BOX

Janet is a middle-aged self-employed woman living in Northern Ireland. She has always found the winter months difficult: "Part of it is being so far north here. In December it gets dark by 3:30 p.m. and it doesn't get light until 9 a.m. There's very little sunlight, so quite often we're in a half-light some of the time." Janet also suffers from episodes of depression, generally triggered by "stress and a lot of things happening at once; I would definitely be more susceptible to that kind of thing." She has found that these episodes tend to happen in winter. "In summer, I feel that I have generally so much more energy. There's so much more light here in summer. It'll be getting light at 3:30 in the morning and from June 22 on, with good weather, it can be light until midnight or so.

"I'd been complaining to a friend about feeling washed-out and having an utter lack of energy. I'd get to December or January and I'd feel the urge to hibernate. People had talked to me about light boxes and I'd thought, *I wonder what that's like?*" She admits that the reported expense of up to £200 (about two hundred and sixty dollars) was a deterrent, but, at a friend's urging, did some research online and found an inexpensive model that could still deliver 10,000 lux.

Janet has now had two winters with her light box and says, "It hasn't transformed my personality, but it has made a perceptible difference when I work at the computer. I found that particularly this past winter, as I had a project and I had six weeks of getting up in the morning, including at the weekends, and working a straight ten- to twelve-hour day in front of a screen. Normally, I would find this difficult. As it will be getting dark, I might be thinking that I don't want to do anything, but this was great: I found that it really perked me up and gave me mental energy."

Janet followed the instructions for use carefully and found that an hour and a half in the mornings is the ideal formula for her. "I have it in front of me when I'm eating my breakfast and I check e-mails and do a little work before going to the office, partly so I have time to use the light box. You can read, you can eat breakfast . . . you don't have to stop doing everything to use it." She is also careful to get outside during the day to boost her exposure to natural light: "I'm more flexible as I don't have to be in the office at set hours, so I'd definitely try to get out at lunchtime, and if there's any sun, I gravitate toward it."

For Janet, the light box is a success. "With it, I find I have more energy and I sleep better. I would never use it after midday. If I used it later in the afternoon, it might keep me awake! I have better concentration and a brighter mood. That feeling you get in the summer, of being more buoyant. Sometimes I dread winter, so this is a really good way of helping me to manage it."

However, there is no doubting the fact that, while the quality of artificial white-light sources may have improved since the 1980s, when Dr. Rosenthal diagnosed SAD, they still cannot replicate the power and full-spectrum qualities of the sun. Because not only can natural white light, which comes from the sun, be a boon to our mood, it can also do a number of other remarkable things:

UV magic

UV light comes in three broad ranges of increasing intensity: the soft UVA, the medium UVB, and the hard UVC. Ultraviolet light UVC, which forms part of the electromagnetic spectrum, has the ability to disinfect water—a quality harnessed by various solar decontamination units used in off-grid communities, but also increasingly in public water facilities and swimming pools. The way UVC light works is that it destroys the formation of DNA linkages in microorganisms, thus preventing them from reproducing and greatly reducing the harm they can cause. As early as the 1930s and 1940s, American scientists such as Dr. George Miley and Dr. Emmett Knott took this principle one step further, finding efficient ways to irradiate human blood to kill resistant germs or viruses. As antibiotics became more popular, interest in ultraviolet blood irradiation (UBI) lessened and it became "the cure that time forgot." Now, however, with antibiotic-resistant viruses and "superbugs," there is a renewed interest in Miley and Knott's discovery.

UVB can help with many skin disorders, such as eczema and psoriasis, and there have been many great successes in this area. However, the ancient Egyptians understood this long before us. Thousands of years ago, they were using psoralens—compounds found in plants that absorb UV light—in combination with sunlight to treat skin diseases.

However, much of our understanding of the power of UV light comes from the work of the Nobel Prize winner Niels Ryberg Finsen, who was awarded the prize in 1903 "in recognition of his contribution to the treatment of diseases, especially *lupus vulgaris*, with concentrated light radiation, whereby he has opened a new avenue for medical science."[33] Born in the Faroe Islands in 1860, Finsen was something of a late bloomer, as his early lack of academic promise was transformed at university. He first released a series of dramatic studies on the treatment of smallpox and chickenpox, where he exposed patients to red light only, with surprisingly good results. Finsen was able to prove that in this case the decisive factor was that red curtains obstruct all light with short wavelengths. Finsen had been born with a rare metabolic disorder called Niemann-Pick disease that was, in principle, incurable. However, he began to notice a sick old cat basking in the sun every day and seeming to recover remarkably. He was inspired by this and discovered that the solution to his own disorder was to sunbathe, and soon he began to experiment with the new and exciting area of phototherapy.

At the time, coal combustion, along with black clothing and heavy interior design, created perpetual light starvation in many people. These diseases of darkness manifested themselves as the dreadful rickets, with its misshapen body bones—indeed, this disease became known as "the English disease," due to the fact that it was so prevalent in English slums.

Light deficiencies also gave rise to horrible dermal eruptions and, as sunlight was scarce in Copenhagen, Finsen would prescribe extensive irradiation of the skin, first with common sunlight condensed through great water-cooled lenses, then increasingly with electric arc lights focused on the inflamed body parts. He called the short-wave light *actinic* or *chemical*, due to its chemical stimulation and bactericidal qualities. The treatments were quite labor-intensive, and the young girls working for hours with the radiation were commonly known as "light elves," but the final results were excellent, and thousands of patients were saved from death or deformity. Cruel surgery had been the only alternative, so the new light therapy was greeted with wonder. Soon, word spread of Finsen's discoveries, and he began to receive visitors from the English and Russian royal families, who were keen to experience his findings for themselves. As a radical humanist, Finsen did not discriminate between his patients: Everyone was offered the same treatment in the same rooms at the same price. Following the award of the Nobel Prize, soon all major hospitals worldwide would inaugurate Finsen clinics for light treatment.[34]

More recently, the American doctor John Parrish has been instrumental in developing a dermatological treatment called PUVA. In this treatment for a number of conditions, from psoriasis to vitiligo to a form of cancer known as cutaneous T-cell lymphoma, the patient is given psoralens (P) and the skin is then exposed to UVA or long-wave ultraviolet radiation. It is considered to be a very successful treatment because it can be applied over large areas of skin, but there have been concerns about its ability to cause skin aging, so caution is always advised. More recently, a treatment called *narrow-band UVB* has become more popular. It uses a specific wavelength of UVB—311–312nm, or nanometers, to be precise—and psoralens are not required. It's important to consult a doctor if you are researching treatments for conditions like psoriasis: yes, you can use a home treatment unit, but it's important that you do so under medical supervision and that you discuss your needs with your doctor first.

Heliotherapy

As Finsen has shown us, heliotherapy, or phototherapy—that is, the treatment of disease by means of sunlight—has been practiced for thousands of years and has been found to be effective at treating certain conditions. Quite apart from that, we know that the sun makes us *feel* good—who doesn't love the first sun of spring after a long winter? However, we are also very well aware of the dangers of excessive sun exposure, in particular that of skin cancer. We are advised to wear broad-brimmed hats, and to put on sun cream—as the Australian health advice puts it: "Slip, Slop, Slap." This advice, first issued in 1980, to slip on a T-shirt, slop on sunscreen, and slap on a hat, took hold in the Australian imagination, and skin cancer rates, particularly in younger people, declined by 5 percent a year from that point. However, health experts in Australia are now worried about a rise in vitamin D deficiency in that country, and a report in the Melbourne *Age* noted that "several prominent endocrinologists, orthopedic specialists and other experts say the message to cover up has led to vitamin D deficiencies in between 30 percent and 70 percent of the population."[35]

Melanoma, a form of skin cancer, is a horrible reality for those who contract it, of course, but in our rush to don sunscreen, could we be ignoring the many benefits of ultraviolet light? After all, if we hide completely away from sunlight, we'll never grow old enough to develop tumors and may find ourselves with a range of other issues instead. In the same Melbourne *Age* article, the endocrinologist Professor Peter Ebeling, head of Osteoporosis Australia, "has linked the low levels of vitamin D to a massive increase in the number of people being treated in hospitals with osteoporosis-related broken bones—up from a daily average of 177 to 262—in the past six years. It costs the health system $1.9 billion a year to treat them."

What's more, sunlight has also been found to reduce blood pressure, as Professor Martin Feelisch of the University of Southampton discovered. It's all to do with nitrous oxide (NO): "NO, along with its breakdown products, known to be abundant in skin, is involved in the regulation of blood pressure. When exposed to sunlight, small amounts of NO are transferred from the skin to the circulation, lowering blood vessel tone. . . ."[36] There is also evidence to suggest that there is a connection between vitamin D production and "good" cholesterol and insulin. Critically, Professor Feelisch suggests, "these results are significant to the ongoing debate about potential health benefits of sunlight and the role of vitamin D in this process. It may be an opportune time to reassess the risks and benefits of sunlight for human health and to take a fresh look at current public health advice. Avoiding excess sunlight exposure is critical to prevent skin cancer, but not being exposed to it at all, out of fear or as a result of a certain lifestyle, could increase the risk of cardiovascular disease. Perhaps with the exception of bone health, the effects of oral vitamin D supplementation have been disappointing."[37]

So it's clear that some sun exposure is more than an elixir for beautiful skin; for most of us it is our primary source of vitamin D, and, as some experts are noting, it's more effective than dietary supplements. Exposure to the sun affects the hormonal balance of your body in two ways: via the eyes into the brain and directly into the skin. Small, regular amounts of sun exposure have also been found to improve many physical health factors, including cardiac output (the amount of blood pumped by the heart in a minute), the oxygen-carrying capacity of the blood, and sex hormones. Yes—ultraviolet light acts as an aphrodisiac! It will also heighten your resistance to infections, as scientists from Georgetown University Medical Center have discovered in their work on T cells, essential for fighting off infection, production of lymphocytes, and tolerance to stress. Sunlight increases general circulation and improves elimination of accumulated cellular waste products. It is a very efficient detoxifier.[38]

Twenty minutes of sunshine on larger body parts three or four times a week is enough for your body reserves to replenish, but your skin type will be a factor, as will your distance from the equator, what you're wearing, and what parts of you are exposed to the sun's rays (for more on sun intake, see page 72).

Strictly speaking, vitamin D is not a vitamin but a fat-soluble hormone. This is important because, according to the Harvard Medical School, "the sun's energy turns a chemical in your skin into vitamin D3, which is carried to your liver and then your kidneys to transform it to active vitamin D." So if you get enough of the sun's rays during the summer, your body will synthesize and stockpile enough to see you through the winter. It is stored in the liver and in fatty tissues, which will cause a problem if you are obese, because body fat obstinately holds on to vitamin D and doesn't release it efficiently. If we get our vitamin D from the sun, our bodies will regulate our intake naturally. Here's the Harvard Medical School again: "Our vitamin D needs vary with age, body weight, percent of body fat, latitude, skin coloration, season of the year, use of sun block, individual reactions to sun exposure, and our overall health. As a general rule, older people need more vitamin D than younger people, large people need more than small people, fat people need more than skinny people, northern people need more than southern people, dark-skinned people need more than fair-skinned people, winter people need more than summer people, sun-phobes need more than sun worshippers, and ill people may need more than well people."

THE SIX SKIN TYPES

Skin types can be divided into six categories, according to what's known as the Fitzpatrick scale, after the doctor who first examined the skin's reaction to the sun's rays:

The most sensitive skin type is found in people of Celtic or Irish origin. Often pale with a rosy complexion, reddish hair, and blue or green eyes, they are extremely vulnerable to sunshine and will always burn but rarely tan. Although they must be extremely cautious about exposure to the sun, with a lot of care and patience, they can increase their tolerance to sunlight.

The next delicate skin family originates in Scandinavia or northern Europe. These individuals, with fair skin, blue eyes, and blond hair, will burn easily and must be cautious about direct exposure to the sun. Given sufficient time and care, they can build up a minimal tan.

The first middle skin type includes people with roots in the Mediterranean, with chestnut hair, hazel eyes, and light olive complexions. They will gradually develop a nice tan but can at times burn if the process is rushed. This group need not take any special precautions, but of course a sensible approach is needed.

The second intermediate skin group includes people of Latino or Chinese origin, who tan easily with a minimal risk of burning. They have lightly pigmented skin, with brown or black hair and dark irises. These people can handle a certain amount of strong sunshine without any danger.

The first dark skin type includes people originating in Arabia or South Asia, with dark eyes and hair and skin of medium pigmentation. They very seldom burn but always tan deeply. These people are naturally adapted to strong sunlight, and their skin may even become pale if they miss out on sunshine for long periods.

The last and darkest skin family includes individuals coming from Africa or indigenous to Australia, with heavy skin pigmentation, black hair, and dark eyes. They tan very deeply, but this doesn't mean that their risk of skin cancer is zero. However, there is no doubting that people with this skin type need a lot of direct sunlight to maintain a healthy metabolism.

We are all different and have individual reactions to light, but the most important thing is to understand the dynamics of your own skin. Learn about how it reacts to light and recognize its inborn restrictions. Discover what those limits are and learn how much sunlight is suitable for you. Are you dark-skinned or pale? Is your skin tough or tender? How much is enough? Eye color can be a good general indicator of your solar tolerance. Those with pale blue, green, or gray eyes are always at risk, whereas those with dark eyes are usually on the safer side.

The sunbed controversy

I have outlined the risks and the benefits of UV, but what about sunbeds? Quite rightly, much has been made of the dangers of using these.

Sunbeds deliver light in a mixture of typically 95 percent UVA and 5 percent UVB, and nothing else. But the method has gained a bad reputation because this 5 percent UVB is known to cause melanoma. The difference between the light from a sunbed and natural sunlight is that natural sunlight contains many more ingredients, making it balanced and wholesome. Think of sunbeds as white bread and sunshine as wholesome whole grain. It's my view that *used only occasionally and with restraint*, sunbeds do have psychotherapeutic value. Being flooded with and surrounded by huge amounts of light is likely to lift the mood of anyone suffering from heavy winter depression. This might seem like a controversial view, given recent advice and restrictions on sunbed use, but again, the watchwords here are *small doses*. Interestingly, in an opinion piece in the UK newspaper *The Independent*, the oncologist Professor Tim Oliver pointed out that many of the dangers of sunbeds come from their use by those under eighteen, "but a recent study of European melanoma rates found that in Sweden—where sunbed use is strictly regulated and tanning salons are supervised, preventing children from using them and protecting adults from over-exposure—there was less melanoma in sunbed users than in non-users."[39]

It's clear that following years of "shun the sun" guidance, experts are beginning to modify their advice and to suggest that small doses of sun may benefit far more than harm, but before you throw yourself under the sun's rays, here are a few sensible tips.

Sunbathing safety

Be aware of the dangers. Sunlight is a wonderful thing, but not when taken in excess. Burning is never, ever good, and some of us with fairer skin, or indeed particular sensitivities, can get skin rashes and even eczema from the sun. If you suspect that your skin is sensitive, always consult a doctor for advice about sun protection.

Start your tanning slowly and then progressively build up a protective layer of pigmentation. This is particularly important if you visit a foreign country. It's tempting on a sun holiday to absorb every last ray, but it's not advisable. Sunburn is never nice and may expose your skin to later dangers. Early-morning and late-afternoon sun are best. A simple procedure will help you when in doubt: Look at the length of your shadow; if it is shorter than your body, the sun is high and caution is needed.

Winter skin is often in a state of hibernation and busy building up fat layers to protect you from the cold. The poor dermis is totally light-starved and has not seen any real sunshine for months. The slow transition to summer skin must be allowed to take its time, so quick tanning on the first sunny day of spring is not advised, and neither is the shock of a sudden sun-filled holiday!

According to the Vitamin D Council, "your body can produce 10,000 to 25,000 IU of vitamin D in just a little under the time it takes for your skin to begin to burn. You make the most vitamin D when you expose a large area of your skin, such as your back, rather than a small area such as your face or arms."[40] Therefore, you should expose a minimum of 10 percent of your naked skin to sunlight—but be creative and don't just overfeed your face and hands; ideally, the whole body should be irradiated from all sides. This means tanning in the nude whenever possible! Body parts that are permanently enclosed in clothes or shoes are hotbeds for fungi and infections. Sunlight is a perfect skin disinfectant, as it kills many germs and bacteria.

Don't just bake in the sun, but move around to get an even exposure of the skin. Even better, do some physical exercise before you start tanning. The improved circulation will stimulate the natural flow of perspiration. Genuine sweat contains an array of substances that help protect your skin, such as salts, fats, and hormones—all tailor-made by your own glands to suit your skin type. Don't remove them with soap before sunbathing.

SUNSCREEN ESSENTIALS

Those of us who were alive during the 1970s will remember the prevalence of tanning oils, but nowadays they are a no-no, because they increase the temperature of your skin and contribute to passive burning. It's also true that there are many less-than-satisfactory, even dubious sunscreens on the market. So what do you need to be aware of when buying and using sunscreen?

- Avoid "once-a-day" sunscreens. According to tests carried out by the consumer organization Which?, a number of sunscreens, including those by "reputable" brands, offered considerably less protection after two hours' sun exposure. The tests revealed that "after six to eight hours of wear, the average protection factor in a sun cream would fall by 74 percent, so that an SPF30, say, would fall to an SPF8."[41]

- Choose your sunscreen carefully. In the EU, sunscreens must be comprised of one-third UVA filters, but this might not apply to sun products bought online. You need to look for an SPF of 30 and a UVA rating of at least four stars as a guide.

- Apply your sunscreen every couple of hours— more if you are swimming. As we learned in chapter 3, sunscreens that advertise themselves as "waterproof" are misleading. If you are swimming, reapply your sunscreen when you get out of the water.

- Apply generously and don't forget those hard-to-reach areas, like the back of the neck, behind the ears, and the lower back. How much? According to experts, "the general rule is a teaspoon for the face, each arm, each leg, the front of the body and the back—that's roughly 35ml of sun cream for the entire body."[42]

- And when the summer is over, ditch the cream. Many of us use the same sunscreen year after year, but it won't be as effective after two weeks in the sun, or indeed after a year in the back of a cupboard. Invest in a fresh bottle regularly. Yes, it may be more expensive, but safety counts when it comes to sun exposure.

- After sun exposure and once you have cleansed your skin, you can use pure aloe vera gel to soothe and moisturize.

Remember, your skin will tan even if you are sitting in the shade. Sunlight bounces around a lot, and the reflected light scatter may suffice to get you started. Sit under a tree or parasol if you have a delicate, pale complexion. Light also penetrates white clothes of loosely woven fabric so you can get a reasonable tan without having to undress at all. A white T-shirt, for example, has an SPF of 4.

Sunlight radiates not only ultraviolet light for tanning but also huge volumes of warming infrared. In hot countries, over-heating of the body can be a very critical issue, as high temperatures can cause heatstroke and dehydration. Always drink plenty of cooling fresh water—and drink it before you start getting parched. If you have been sweating profusely, extra salt may be needed to replace lost minerals.

FOOD AND DRINK FOR SUN WORSHIPPERS

When living and tanning under a strong sun, you might be surprised by which foods and drinks work to keep you cool. Some researchers have actually found that drinking a hot drink might keep you cool, as the sweat you produce evaporates and your body cools down![43] More to the point, many cold drinks contain a lot of sugar, so plain, not-too-cold water is best for thirst—sweet and sticky ice creams will only exacerbate your thirst and make your head spin. And go easy on the alcohol. Getting drunk in the heat of the day will seriously upset your brain and will also dehydrate you. Follow the example of people who live in hot climates—they eat hot, spicy foods for a reason. Those antimicrobials will keep food poisoning at bay, but, more to the point, all that spice makes you sweat, and, in a hot climate, sweating is good for you. "Gustatory facial sweating" might not sound like a pleasant side effect of eating spicy chili, but it works!

If you are going skiing or hiking at a high altitude—take care. Ultraviolet light is much more intense at higher altitudes because there is less intervening air to absorb it. The highland air feels fresh and invigorating on the skin, but the UV burns will come later, so take extra precautions. Also, if you are basking on a beach, a cooling seaside breeze can be very deceptive and could well fool you into underestimating the strength of the sun. Children in particular love splashing and playing around in the water, but their little bodies are very susceptible to burning, so try to make sure they dry off regularly, and protect their skin by reapplying sunscreen frequently.

THINK LOCAL

The weather around the world is as diverse as the human race itself. Use your common sense and learn how to live happily with the sun. The air is normally clearer and cooler in the morning than in the evening, and the light is shifted slightly toward the blue and ultraviolet range. The same logic applies to seasons but on a larger scale. The atmospheric layers are clearer after the cold of winter and facilitate the passage of ultraviolet light. In early autumn, the air is filled with dust, pollen, and humidity after the fertile summer season. This filters out the high frequencies and gives the light a reddish appearance. Pre-noon tanning in the early days of summer would therefore be the optimal strategy for catching the rays of natural UV without undue heat.

THE DEPTHS OF RED

The last "super light" on our agenda is infrared, or IR. First discovered by the astronomer William Herschel in 1800, IR has been of immense benefit medically. But before we look at just what a wonder it is, let's return to our electromagnetic spectrum. If we remember that only a small part of this spectrum is visible to us, well, IR falls beyond the visible spectrum with longer waves than those of visible light, and even though we can't see it, we can "feel" it as heat. The most important source of IR is sunlight. Other common sources include heaters, saunas, motors, and cars, as well as ovens and irons.

DID YOU KNOW THAT?

- Certain snakes, such as rattlesnakes, use infrared "imaging" to detect warm-blooded prey.
- Fish use near infrared to orient themselves while swimming.
- Night-vision goggles use infrared technology.

- The earliest microwaves weren't actually microwaves at all, but "infrared ovens." You'll also find infrared sensors used in kitchen thermometers.[44]
- Security lights use infrared technology to detect the heat coming from people or objects.

However, our interest in IR is primarily therapeutic, and one such effect of infrared light is improved blood flow during wound healing. The enhanced circulation increases the supply of proteins, nutrients, water, and oxygen to the affected areas and assists in the elimination of toxic cellular waste products. Infrared irradiation is used for a large number of common symptoms—arthritis, bruises, cramps, inflammations, migraines, sprains, tennis elbow: No wonder it's a favorite tool of sports medicine. Where IR really comes into its own is with pain. In a trial conducted by the Rothbart Center for Pain Care in North York, Ontario, patients with a back pain score of 6.9 out of a possible 10 found this reduced to a 3 after a course with IR pads. (This compared with a placebo group who went from 7.4 to 6.)[45]

There are a huge number of IR devices on the market now, promising to treat everything from sunburn to weight loss, and even to cure hair loss, so it's important to do your research. For example, the National Center for Health Research, in Washington, DC, found that there was no link between weight loss and IR technology,[46] although a study of infrared light on skin treatments found that "treatment with IR radiation may be an effective and safe non-ablative remodeling method of the skin, and it may have some use as a supportive method in the treatment of photo-aged skin."[47] Infrared therapy has also been said to help to stimulate hair regrowth. You will notice that there are a large number of IR brushes and combs that promise scalp health, but again, do your research. Pick a device that has been approved by the appropriate body.

What about IR saunas? Perhaps you'll have heard some of the claims about their benefits, but what's the difference between an IR and a conventional sauna? Well, the IR sauna is a lot cooler than the traditional Finnish one: about 40 degrees compared to the latter's 80 degrees. Conventional saunas heat you by heating the air around you, so that you sweat. Infrared saunas heat you, but don't heat the air around you: You still sweat, but it may be more tolerable if you don't like the intense heat of a sauna. As to the health benefits, well, some smaller studies[48] have reported improvements in people with rheumatoid arthritis, but as yet no large-scale studies have been completed. However, what is clear is that IR saunas will do no harm and provide a pleasant alternative to the traditional sauna.

THE MAGIC OF BLUE

In chapter 4, we learned about avoiding blue light at night due to its overstimulating effects and potential to damage the eyes, but light in the wavelength range of 415–495nm (that we see as a range from cyan to violet) has potent super qualities that merit our attention. The effects range from antibacterial action to liver support, and may be more or less pronounced depending on the wavelength of blue light used. At the shorter end of blue, near the violet (400–415nm), the effects are more antibacterial but with little penetration of the skin. This is beneficial in treating the bacteria associated with acne, as well as nasty hospital bugs such as MRSA. High-frequency blue light is a stimulant for many body tissues, but the energy overload can also harm the retina.

At the longer end of the blue range (450–490nm), there is deeper penetration of the skin with less antibacterial action. These longer wavelengths of blue light can interact with the blood in the capillaries, neutralizing toxins as it passes through. This action is utilized in treating liver disorders such as neonatal jaundice and Crigler-Najjar syndrome, which are caused by the body's failure to break down the metabolic waste product bilirubin. The method was accidentally discovered by British nurses during the London Blitz, when hospitals were evacuated into churches and country manors. Babies sleeping under blue stained-glass windows inexplicably recovered from jaundice.

A less commonly known application of blue light is in the treatment of hyperpigmentation or age-related dark spots. These arise when fine brownish pigment granules called lipofuscin spontaneously deposit in the skin, particularly under exposure to the ultraviolet rays of strong sunlight. Many people find these spots to be an aesthetic nuisance—but they can be treated. Focused blue light will be absorbed by the lipofuscin molecules, causing the pigment patches to eventually dry up and fade.

How can you personally benefit from the magic of blue? Just like infrared, blue light is now harnessed in devices for home use. The most common usage is for skin complaints such as acne or psoriasis. Blue light kills acne bacteria quickly and naturally, without side effects, while in cases of psoriasis, it has a regulatory action on skin-cell production and inflammation. Blue light is gentler than PUVA and has none of the skin-damaging effects of ultraviolet light. Similarly, exposure to blue light can help with mood or sleep disorders when natural daylight comes at a premium, for example, in the depths of a Nordic winter or for a hospital worker on the night shift. Examples of blue-light devices available for home use include blue LED facial devices or lamps for acne treatment (note that when treating the face with blue light, eye protection is essential); portable blue-light boxes for the treatment of SAD or winter blues; small wearable devices for psoriasis treatment; and blue LED oral devices and toothbrushes for gum health and tooth whitening.

Today, many of us in the developed world are aware of the benefits of a healthy lifestyle. Remember, too, at the start of our adventure, we mentioned the brain's ability to literally eat shining photons? It uses light as natural software, and a therapeutic light dose can help it perform on a superior level. This might be particularly advantageous when studying for an important exam, preparing for a sports competition, or embarking on a creative endeavor. Indeed, the super lights can enhance our well-being on many levels, from the purely biological to the abstract psychological. How then to tap into them?

As I mentioned in chapter 1, in the 1980s Professor Tiina Karu in Moscow found that monochromatic light can replicate the biological effects of the miraculous laser—most notably in the repair of damaged DNA. The human eye–brain is highly sensitive to light and also attracted to beauty, so in my own practice I always used the pretty mono-light for psychotherapeutic treatments. The light was in the visual range (400–700nm) and diffused into 3-D to create an illusion of floating. There were no set rules but clients could freely choose the colors they desired. A full-light dose was complete in ten minutes, and for most cases one session a month was sufficient.

In my view, concentrated light works like a photonic vaccine, where small doses work wonders. Remember—LLLT stands for "low-level laser therapy." As casual research will show, there are any number of light therapies on offer, and finding what works for you depends on what you are looking for. If you seek an improvement in mood, light therapy has proven benefits. If you have a skin issue such as psoriasis, you may well have tried light therapy to alleviate the condition. Light therapies are also available for treating conditions such as allergic rhinosinusitis, although treatment is expensive, so you may need to weigh the potential benefits against the costs.

Whichever way you choose to explore the world of the super lights, there is just one guiding principle: Have respect for their potency. View them more like a shot of concentrated photons than a square meal of everyday sunlight. So whether you are trying a device for home use or consulting a professional therapeutic light practitioner, pay attention to the advice and recommendations for usage. Just as you would adhere to the dosage of a high-potency vitamin pill, you should adhere to the dosage of high-potency therapeutic light. There is detailed information about various colored-light treatments and their effects in the Color Gallery in the appendix on page 139, which can guide you on your personal discovery of the super lights.

EYE FITNESS

Vision is the art of seeing what is invisible to others.

—JONATHAN SWIFT

Of course, that great satirist Jonathan Swift was talking about insight, about noticing what others might not see, but his statement reminds me of the importance of looking after your eyesight. This may seem a bit of a contradiction—after all, if you have, say, short sight, or if you have inherited an astigmatism, there's not a lot you can do about it, but while the idea of "natural vision correction" might be controversial, what's perfectly clear is that our eyes have to do a lot of work in daily life. As our windows to the world, they have to detect and decipher colossal amounts of information—and with our increasing reliance on screens, looking after your eyesight is more important than ever.

Before we talk about how to improve eye health, let's have a look at how our eyes actually function in harmony with our brains to process visual information.

THE EYES

We humans have our eyes mounted frontally on our faces, with
a generous overlap of both visual fields. This is how most predators view the world. Our two eyes observe our surroundings
from slightly different angles and each eye receives a slightly
different input. You can see this very simply if you first close
one eye, then the other. We can judge distance well, but we lack
a wide-angle perspective. Prey animals are another story. Their
eyes are mounted on the sides of their heads, and rabbits, for
example, can see a full panorama of 360 degrees. This makes
sense, of course, because they can graze happily while keeping
an eye out for predators.

The Eyelids

Our eyes are covered by our eyelids, mobile and elastic structures that act like soft shutters to mechanically protect the eyeball and prevent an excessive influx of light. They also guard
the outer cornea and moisten the delicate inner optics through
frequent blinking.

The Muscles

The eyeball is externally controlled by six pairs of surprisingly
strong muscles fitted around its rim: two pairs for doing vertical
scans, two pairs for making horizontal sweeps, and two pairs for
performing complex rotatory movements. Like the muscles in
the rest of the body, these six muscle bundles constantly initiate
and execute complex motion patterns. When observing interesting objects, our eyes will incessantly change focus without us
noticing. They quickly skip back and forth to cover all salient

points of the scenery. These ocular jumps are called *saccades*, and they must be perfectly coordinated with the general motion of body and head.

The eyes perform three kinds of different movements to register external events:

- ‣ Slow sweeps for continual update.

- ‣ Speedy jumps 5 times per second.

- ‣ Random tremors 50 times per second.

The Pupil

The pupil is the gateway to the inner eye and opens or closes according to external light levels. This reflex controls the quantity of incoming light, but our pupils' reactions to light and darkness aren't the same. The pupil closes much faster than it opens and automatically adjusts itself to strong light within seconds; however, its adaptation to darkness is much slower—it can take up to an hour. Interestingly, our pupils have also been shown to react in the absence of stimuli: Bruno Laeng and Unni Sulutvedt, two Swedish scientists, conducted an experiment in which they invited subjects to look at a series of triangles, which were variously brightly or dimly lit. The subjects' pupils reacted as expected, widening for the dimly lit objects and narrowing for the brightly lit ones. However, Laeng and Sulutvedt then requested that their subjects simply imagine the same shapes: their pupils did exactly the same thing, even though they weren't looking at anything! A fascinating glimpse into the world of neuroscience.[49]

The Eyeball

The eyeball isn't a ball, of course, but almost a sphere, fitting neatly into our eye sockets. The front of the eyeball, consisting of the cornea and anterior chamber, is comprised of static tissue, but the cornea protects the rest of the eye from dust and bacteria and refracts incoming light onto the lens. The cornea provides the lion's share—about 70 percent—of the eye's optical power. The transparent protein lens controls the direction and focus of the incoming light and is suspended by fine ciliary muscle fibers that regulate its curvature.

The interior ocular cavity is filled with a transparent jelly called the vitreous body, which protects the millions of photosensitive cells in the retina. Behind it lies the light-absorbing retina, where the incoming photons are trapped and their energy is converted into electric nerve signals, to be forwarded into the visual centers of the brain. The retina measures only a quarter of a millimeter in thickness but has the highest blood flow and oxygen consumption of the entire body. This complex tissue consists of light-sensitive nerve cells sandwiched in three layers, which are ultimately bundled together into the optic nerve. The optic nerve leaves the eyeball via the optic disc.

Interestingly, the optic disc has no light-receptor cells—it's your blind spot. Vertebrates have a blind spot, but octopi, for example, do not. If you'd like to test your blind spot, draw a small, shaded circle on the left side of a piece of paper. Draw a plus sign at a distance of 12 cm (5 inches) to the right. Hold the piece of paper about 20 cm (8 inches) from your eye and focus your left eye on the plus sign. Now, gradually bring the piece of paper closer to your eye, still focusing on the plus sign—what happens? At a certain point, the dot will disappear! Now, reverse the process and look at the dot with your right eye . . . and so on. Fascinating!

The central pit, or fovea, of the retina is located on the optical axis of the eye. This tiny depression measures only a millimeter across and is densely packed with cone cells, cone-shaped cells that can discriminate the color composition of the incoming light. Visual acuity is at its height here, and this is where we fix our gaze for detailed observation. The foveal cones lie exactly on the focal point of the lens, and this makes them vulnerable to piercing light of high frequency. As an initial protection, the sensitive cone cells are covered by a shielding yellow filter called the macula lutea.

The periphery of the retina is an older and less specialized ocular structure. Most blue color cones and all the dark-sensitive rods are distributed on this outer edge. This is why our peripheral vision has really poor resolution and cannot detect any detail but is still vital to survival. These peripheral parts are keenly aware of general background motion and rapid motion change. If something calls for extra scrutiny, the eye will then adjust for a sharp focus. Without a well-functioning peripheral field, we have what we call *tunnel vision*.

The rods in our retinas are adapted for supersensitive nocturnal vision, and while we can see minute amounts of light thanks to the 100 million rods, it is a slow process. Our animal companions have many more rod cells, because many of them need better night vision to hunt.

Meanwhile, the color-coding cones are busy during bright daylight or full sun. We have about 5 million small pointed cones for advanced color perception. Coding speed and precision levels are much higher than with the rods, and cones are active in three portions of the spectrum, commonly called *red*, *green,* and *blue.* That doesn't mean that we see only red, green, and blue, of course: It's a complicated process, but the overlap of cones and the signals the brain receives allows us to see other colors. People who are "color-blind" or "color deficient" are thought to have faulty color cones, or possibly the signal to the brain is not working properly.

The rods and cones send incoming nerve signals to one million ganglion cells that collect and transmit electro-pulses to the brain. The ganglion cells cannot see or detect any physical objects as such, but recent research has shown that some of them have optical sensitivity. They decode the general coloring of the ambient light and then "entrain" the circadian rhythms of the body. Our cycles of wakefulness and sleep are largely controlled by this newly detected group of photosensitive cells.

THE BRAIN

Of course, seeing isn't only done by the eyes. It is estimated that some 90 percent of the visual process occurs inside the brain. Therefore, while "seeing" is a physical process, perception is largely a psychological process, of which culture and expectation form a large part. We can only see what we expect to see—the unknown is invisible to the mind.

The primary visual center, known as V1 or *substantia nigra,* is the most investigated area of the visual cortex, which is found in the occipital lobe in the back of the head. It is found among many animals as well. It seems to act as a central relay, where incoming impulses are sorted for further specialized analysis. V2 will compare finely graded structures and establish neural pathways of visual association. Above and slightly in front of the first pair we find region V3, which provides a broad view of the total visual input to allow the eye to interpret global motion. Below V1 is sector V4, where simple geometric forms are examined and the dimension of color comes alive. Zone V5 lies beneath the ears and has a special bearing with its own nerve conduits. It receives direct impulses from the retina and guides the motor activity of the eyes into a smooth flow. Below this motor area sits a sixth region, named the *inferior temporal gyrus*, which has a capacity to recognize multifaceted objects and faces.

EYESIGHT AND EVOLUTION

It is interesting to note that, for example, the Aboriginal people of Australia have eyesight that can be up to four times better than that of non-Aboriginal people. The reason for this is thought to be evolutionary: To survive in the outback, poor sight would have been a distinct disadvantage. Professor Hugh Taylor describes it thus: "[For] a hunter-gatherer, good vision, to be able to see a kangaroo lying in the shade, or find a waterhole or whatever, would be critically important. Bad vision is a really bad thing to have if you are trying to survive in those areas."[50] Sadly, because of many other factors, Aboriginal people are much more likely to suffer from eye problems in later life, and this is also the case for many people in the developing world, who do not have access to treatment for common eye diseases, or, indeed, such conditions as myopia.

Myopia is an inherited condition, but research has shown that nearsightedness can be affected by the amount of time outdoors, which might explain why some populations have better distance vision than others. A study comparing Chinese children living in Australia and those living in Singapore or China found that the Australian children had better distance vision, probably because they spent more time outdoors. A review for the American Academy of Ophthalmology, quoted in the *Daily Telegraph*, found that the prevalence of shortsightedness in some countries might indeed have to do with the populace's reading more, but that "it might be something to do with relaxing the focusing mechanism in the eye and returning it to normal distance vision, and the wavelengths of light we are exposed to outside could also have an impact," as Professor Paul Foster explained.[51]

And now, armed with detailed knowledge of our eyes and brain and how they process visual information, it's time to get them working! Using your eye muscles will maintain healthy ocular elasticity and blood flow throughout your life. Maintaining eye fitness is not a new idea; it was advocated a hundred years ago by the American doctor William Bates. He discovered the medical properties of the famous stress hormone adrenaline and found that nervous schoolchildren often had inferior vision. His remedy was a series of simple eye movements specially designed to strengthen the ocular muscles. Today we would call his method *eye yoga*.

Dr. Bates claimed to have helped thousands of clients regain their natural vision, but scientific rigor was different a hundred years ago. Nonetheless, one thing still remains certain: Human eyes never evolved to be used under electric lighting. Unnatural light can, in my view, wreak havoc on the eyes, and I can only speak from personal experience. I spent my entire youth wearing glasses, and eventually the situation just got worse. But at the age of forty I started practicing the Bates method of eye yoga, and my eyesight gradually improved. Now, at the age of seventy, I can read perfectly well without any glasses.

You will have to make up your own minds, but eye yoga is relaxing, invigorating, and enjoyable, and there is no harm at all in keeping your eye muscles in tip-top shape, particularly in a world that presents our eyes with so many challenges.

EYE YOGA

Before we start

Let's begin by relaxing our bodies. Move your body from side to side like in a slow dance. Shift your weight from one leg to the other and learn to play with the elasticity of the body posture. You may want to put on some music.

Next, stand on your tiptoes and find a position where you are in dynamic balance. No problems? Really easy? Now close your eyes and notice what happens to your stance. Suddenly, keeping your balance becomes maddeningly difficult, and most of us will stumble in just a few seconds. The body desperately needs to see the outer world in order to navigate. Try to build an inner center of gravity from where you can start to stabilize. The yoga pose known as "tree" is good for balance, but it takes practice, so try it using a wall for support in the first instance. *Yoga Journal* suggests the following: Stand straight with your heels together, your right side about half an arm's length from the wall. Raise the right arm and place the right hand on the wall for support. Shift your weight onto the right leg, and on an inhalation bend the left leg, bringing the foot to the inner thigh. Keep the right leg firm and both hips facing forward. Lengthen both sides of the waist equally. Take five to ten deep breaths before practicing on the other side. After a time, you can take your hand away from the wall. Obviously, be careful if you have any injuries or issues that might affect your balance.

Shoulder roll

Move your shoulders up and down and in all possible directions, to loosen up tight tendons and ligaments around the upper chest. This will ensure an improved blood flow to the eye–brain system. Get someone to massage your neck and shoulders if needed. Now, move and turn your head around in a circular motion to soften the neck muscles: They easily contract from stress and lack of motion. A colossal number of nerves, arteries, and lymph vessels pass through the neck. Try lowering your head as far as you can toward your chest. Now, roll your head slowly to the left, then in a circular motion up to the ceiling, then down to the right, before bringing it to rest toward your chest again. Repeat this motion a number of times—but be gentle!

Palming

Sit down comfortably and relax. Close your eyes and gently hold each eyeball, grasping around it with your fingertips. Give it a softly rolling massage to prepare for the muscle training. Next, cup both hands tightly over the eyes without touching the eyes. Make sure no external light can enter around the rim. Enjoy the soothing darkness combined with the warmth of your hands. This technique is known as palming. Sit in this way for as long as you like. As an alternative, place your palms over your open eyes, then gently close them.

The Exercises

You will be surprised at how demanding these exercises are. After a session of eye yoga you will be openly yawning and want to go to sleep, but once you have practiced a couple of times it will all become easier. We'll begin with some stretches.

Stretch up

First, look upward without tilting your head back to compensate, and find a spot on the ceiling onto which to fix your gaze. When you have reached your limit, stay there for a while but then slowly extend the range a little farther and a little farther until your eyebrows seem to get in the way. Initially, the muscles will feel tight, but eventually they will let go. The feeling of muscles stretching is a very special sensation. First you will feel a firm resistance, but keep applying some pressure—suddenly you will experience a loose feeling of relaxation when the muscles ease. Take it easy and find the place where they open up. When everything feels soft, look straight ahead. Firmly close and open the eyes a couple of times to lubricate them.

Stretch down

Now do the same thing looking straight down as far as you can. Focus on the navel area without bending your neck. This is usually a lot easier. We are much more accustomed to looking down while reading and working. Hold your gaze until you get that sensation of muscular softness, then look straight ahead again. Firmly close and open the eyes as before.

Vertical sweep

Now that your vertical eye muscles are fully prepared and stretched, it's time to perform full sweeping movements. Look up as far as possible and then immediately look down as far as you can. Repeat this cycle fourteen times, making the sweeps large and generous. Then blink and breathe. In fact, don't forget to breathe! Some people concentrate so hard that they forget and subconsciously hold their breath.

Stretch right

Next come the horizontal muscles. Fix your gaze on a point as far right as you can and keep looking at it *without turning your head*. Extend your range a little farther and still a bit more. Go for it. This is an unusual experience, and other parts of the face will want to join in. Be patient and wait for that sudden phase of soft relaxation. Then look ahead and blink firmly.

Stretch left

As above, but this time to the left. Wait for the smooth extension of the eye muscles to occur and then look ahead. Then do some vigorous blinking.

Horizontal sweep

Your horizontal eye muscles have now been fully stretched, so it's time to give them a real workout. Sweep right and left in fourteen full cycles. Try to do this with as broad a reach as you can, ensuring you cover the entire visual range. Look to the front and blink.

Diagonal stretch, upper right

Now for some quite difficult directions. The diagonals involve several muscle pairs working simultaneously. Find a point in the upper right-hand corner of your visual field, at the very limit of your capacity. Fix your gaze on it and slowly stretch a bit farther and a bit farther. Facial muscles are likely to join in a slow dance. When ready, look ahead and blink.

Diagonal stretch, lower left

Do the same as before but in the opposite direction. Looking to the lower left is usually easy. In daily life, your eyes are used to looking downward. Remember to blink once you have finished.

Diagonal sweep

Now that you have nicely extended your diagonal reach, it's time to make the full sweep, from upper right to lower left, fourteen times. Don't forget to blink at the end.

Diagonal stretch, upper left

Like its counterpart upper right, this is a difficult direction, as such high-reaching slanted positions are rarely employed in daily life. Upper diagonals are often connected with muscular spasms and subconscious emotions. Blink for a while and relax the eye muscles after the stretch.

Diagonal stretch, lower right

Stretch diagonally downward to the lower right-hand corner
of your visual field. This direction may feel quite familiar and
should be easy to perform. Finish off by blinking.

Diagonal sweep

Your eye muscles are now elastic and ready for the sweeping movements, this time from upper left to lower right. Make the same
large trajectories as before. Pause to blink once you are finished.

Your eye muscles are remarkably strong, but for many of you they
have been dormant for half a lifetime. By now you may be quite
exhausted but also strangely elated. Take a look around the room
and notice the difference. Perhaps everything looks brighter or
your visual field looks larger. But this is just a first step. We will
now calibrate your wonderful eye muscles for precision work.

Circles

The first time you do this exercise, it helps if you have an assis-
tant standing in front of you with a bright object in their hand,
such as a colored ball. The ball is slowly rotated in a large circle
and you follow it with your eyes as best you can. Very few of us
can make perfect circles, and your eyes will want to take sudden
shortcuts. Note where deviations from the perfect circle occur.
This is where your tight muscles need extra training. Eventually,
you will be able to do the perfect circle without help. Do eight
rounds both ways and take extra time on the difficult sections.
A little blinking is always recommended.

Complex shapes

Circles are elementary shapes and very good for correcting simple deviations. But visual life isn't that simple, and you should now aim to extend your range of movement to include many other geometric forms. Figure eights are the next logical step. They involve much more motor control of the eyes and are more difficult to perform. Try to experiment with both vertical and horizontal orientations. Again, notice where your eyes want to tense up and make erratic jumps. Where are your weak directions? Give them some extra attention.

The next level of geometric complexity involves free shapes, and you will find these everywhere in nature. Carefully allow your hungry eyes to trace the finely serrated outlines of maple and oak leaves, for example.

ZOOMING

We have now trained your outer eye muscles. Next up are the inner ciliary muscles that surround and suspend the lens. When fully active, they can adjust its curvature and give you a decent zoom. Walk outdoors into an expanse with an open view. You will be exercising your depth perception and must be able to see objects at far distances. Treetops will do, mountain peaks are better, and clouds are really good. A full moon is best of all. It will train your eyes to operate at an extended focus. The moon is the most distant object, with surface details that are plainly visible to the naked eye.

Hold out your hand and raise a finger, then firmly fix your gaze on the fingertip. Really focus both eyes on the fingertip and don't let them stray. Then let them jump to a distant object and fix on that. Zoom back and forth for ten full cycles, giving yourself time to get the focus sharp. This sequence can be further elaborated with several intermediate steps: Gaze at your fingertip; focus on the treetop; spot the nocturnal cloud; admire the lunar craters; then look back to your fingertip again.

This core program, originated by Dr. Bates, can be supplemented with many more interesting eye movements. Get to know your own vision and pay attention to movements you find more difficult. You may have to work on these aspects a little more. Most important, keep it simple and stick to a regular program. Take a few minutes every now and then. Use spare moments to let the eyes have some fun and play around. You can do the exercises at home, in the office, or on a bus or airplane if you are feeling brave—yes, performing eye exercises really makes you look ridiculous!

MORE EYESIGHT-ENHANCING TECHNIQUES

Use color to enhance your vision

In *green light*, the normal eye will focus the image perfectly on the retina, giving you the experience of a clear image. This made biological sense for forest-dwelling apes and hominids, for whom green was the standard backdrop. Green lies in the middle of the visible spectrum and has often been used as a background for visually demanding tasks such as reading. Many blackboards used to be green, and so were school desks and things like computer circuit boards, where visual acuity is crucial. So if your vision is normal, use green in some form to stabilize your gaze.

In *red light*, the image will focus behind the retina and your brain will interpret this as a blurry image. If you happen to be nearsighted or myopic, the eyes will want to place the focal point in front of the retina. With a bit of luck, these two errors will cancel each other out and the outcome may be a reasonably sharp picture. Thus, a red table or reading lamp may be helpful if you are nearsighted.

In *blue light*, exactly the opposite happens, and the image will now focus in front of the retina. But farsighted, or hyperopic, eyes want to project the sharp focus behind the retinal plane. Here again we have a neat compromise where two natural inaccuracies can annul each other. A blue desk or office lamp may be ideal if you have farsighted eyes.

Wobbly reading

Reading in a shaky bus or subway train may be uncomfortable, but it is a particularly good exercise for your advanced ocular motor coordination. Counteracting the rattle and wobble demands a lot of neuronal fine-tuning and is excellent for maintaining the coordinated focus of both eyes.

Eye rinse

We are creatures of the ocean, and the eyes are particularly watery. Give them regular splashes to replenish the supply. Use hot or cool sterile water (water that has been boiled first, then allowed to cool down) according to taste, and possibly add a pinch of salt. Also make a habit of blinking every so often. Weeping for joy is also recommended. Tears are antiseptic and will moisturize the corneas, and will keep your eyes clear of irritating dust and pollutants. The added liquid will also act as a lens coating and boost their refractive power.

———————

So there you have it, the fascinating eye in a nutshell. Whether you have perfect vision or not, I hope you enjoyed the stimulating exercises and that they helped you to see the world in a new and refreshing way.

LIGHTING IN THE HOME

A dark house is always an unhealthy house.

—FLORENCE NIGHTINGALE

When Nightingale said this, she was referring to the dark and gloomy conditions of houses in Victorian England. She continued by talking about how the "want of light promotes scrofula [a disease connected to TB] and rickets among the children," which was certainly true in the nineteenth century. Nowadays, our "want of light" is part of life, with so many of us living indoors, due to work and schooling, but it's also a lifestyle choice: With so much to occupy us indoors, why venture outside?

Well, we need to improve our connection with the outside world, for a start. There's no doubting that it affects our mental and physical well-being. According to a study carried out by Dutch scientists in 2007 for the *Journal of Epidemiology & Community Health*, people who lived within a kilometer [half a mile] of a woodland or park suffered from less anxiety and depression;[52] while a Swedish study found that runners who ran in open parkland were brighter and happier than those who exercised in the gym. The "Green Gym" movement run by the Conservation Volunteers in the UK offers the opportunity for people to go outdoors and do conservation activities such as planting, weeding, and clearing in the name of conservation—but also to be in the outdoors with other people and get some exercise. Some GPs have even begun to prescribe Green Gym sessions to patients who need to get fit. If there isn't a Green Gym near you, why not find a community garden to volunteer in, or start an outdoor community project of your own?

If this wasn't proof enough of the benefits of nature, according to the University of Rochester, being close to nature can make you a better person, too. In a number of experiments, volunteers were exposed to either natural or man-made settings and set a series of tasks. In one experiment, volunteers were given £5 (around seven dollars) and told they could either keep it for themselves or donate it to another volunteer, who would be given an extra £5. Fascinatingly, the "nature" control group proved to be the more generous![53]

However, after singing the praises of nature, we must remember that the subject of this chapter is lighting in the home. My point is that it should be our goal to be outdoors as much as possible, but for many of us, particularly those of us who live in northern climes, it is understood that we will spend a lot of time indoors in the winter—which is why there is so much attention in my native Sweden to home design. Swedish architects have long understood the necessity of opening our houses to light, and of incorporating light-maximizing features such as large windows and clever spaces, as well as an interior palette that makes the most of whatever light we have. I am finding this to be the case in a project I am currently developing with a colleague, Kjell Wallin. Facing south is always a premium, but offices with large windows can get very hot in summer, so most industrial windows have a surface coating to block incoming infrared heat. But there is a catch—this filter also blocks color perception, and rooms take on a gloomy look, where human faces appear sallow. I am currently working with Kjell to develop office windows with higher light transmission and natural color rendering.

Swedish architects have long understood the necessity of opening our houses to light, and of incorporating light-maximizing features such as large windows and clever spaces, as well as an interior palette that makes the most of whatever light we have.

HOME BUILDS

If you are lucky enough to be building your own home, or to be buying a modern home, look out for the following.

The *orientation* of the house, and indeed the rooms within it, to the sun. As the modernist architect Louis Kahn put it, "The sun never knew how great it was until it hit the side of a building." Orientation to the sun has been the watchword of buildings from ancient Greece to the present day. It makes sense to have your living space open to the sun, at the expense of your bedrooms, in which you'll spend less of your time.

We all look for south-facing, but this isn't always possible, so look for spaces that can be "opened up" to let light in. Look at glazing, too. You can be your very own Mies van der Rohe, with a clever choice in glazing. Mies was one of the founders of the modernist movement, and with his use of glass and steel created many of the iconic buildings of the twentieth century, such as the Seagram Building, the Barcelona Pavilion, and the Farnsworth House, with its windows on all sides to let the trees that surround it bring nature "in" to the building.[54]

Le Corbusier was also a proponent of using windows with great artistry to let in light and play with it. His Chapelle Notre Dame du Haut in Ronchamp, France, is a master class in using windows to let in light at particular times of the day—and to let it in in magical ways. The windows in his chapel aren't big, but are used in creative ways, with a range of different-size slots cut into the deep stone to give a slightly otherworldly effect, which contributes to the visitor's spiritual experience. On a more practical level, big windows will let in more light, of course, but don't forget skylights, which let in a lovely light, and rooflights. And don't despair as you can now buy rooflights for flat roofs also—and nowadays they are less likely to leak.

Shadows are also very important in your home. There is something about the interplay of shadows and light that is magical, and the reflection of, say, a tree's dappled leaves in your living room will really let nature in. But shadow also adds depth and texture to your space. Imagine if you didn't have shadow—your space would look very flat and one-dimensional.

OLD HOMES

Those of us who live in Victorian homes might find ourselves living with small windows and rooms and gloomy architecture. It's always possible to add a window to let light in, in a hall-way, for example, or to look at a tubular daylight device, some-times called a Solatube, which can light dank basements and hallways with a soft, slightly ghostly glow. You can also put a window in above a door—a transom window might bring in more much-needed light. Or you can look at "opening up" the space by removing interior walls—with the advice of an expert, of course!—by replacing big wooden doors with glass-paneled ones, and by ensuring you don't clutter your windows with fur-niture, books, or decorative items. Unless you are very keen on curtains, consider blinds or shutters, or use light, bright mate-rials if privacy is an issue.

Clean your windows! You'd be surprised how much light is stolen by grubby windows—and steer clear of dark window frames. Somber sills will absorb and steal portions of incoming precious rays, but worst of all they provide a harsh contrast to the brilliance of daylight. The outside is always much, much brighter than the inside, and adjusting between the two lumi-nous extremes is tiresome for your eyes. If necessary, paint existing dark frames in a white or pastel shade. Gloss paint is preferable, as it gives better light reflection than matte. Also, when it comes to a brighter interior, look at light floor tiles or wood, rather than a light-stealing carpet.

Clean your windows! You'd be surprised how much light is stolen by grubby windows— and steer clear of dark window frames.

PLANNING YOUR LIGHT HOME

You can make a big difference in the light quality of your home with well-chosen electric lighting. Again, there are two approaches, according to whether you are building your own home, or if you have to make do with existing sockets and light fittings. Whatever your situation, it pays to have a plan.

Go from room to room and make notes about what happens/ will happen in each. Take the living room, for example—what will you be doing in there? Watching TV, but also reading? Will there be children playing? Might you also use it as a study? If so, you're going to need different kinds of lighting for each purpose. What about lighting paintings, photographs, or ornaments? Moving on to the kitchen, you'll be eating your meals there, but also cooking, so you'll need good light to do your chopping and stirring; and your children may be doing their homework at the kitchen table, so you'll need lighting there as well as for eating. Another thing to consider is the age range in the house; older people need substantially brighter light than youngsters.

Think about the natural light in the room. Do you use this room during the day or only at night? Where does the natural light come in, and what kind of light is it—i.e., south-facing, in which case you'll need to deal with glare; or north-facing, which will need to be "warmed up"? If you live in the Southern Hemisphere, of course, the opposite will apply. East-facing rooms will look lovely in the morning, but dingy by evening, and west-facing will have strong sunlight in the late afternoon.

Now, get your pencil and paper out and draw a plan of your room, marking where the furniture will be and what features are already in place, such as fireplaces and windows. Mark the ceiling height, and which direction the room faces. Remember what each person will be doing in each room. Other things to consider might be the number of switches you'll need. Ideally, you won't want to be flicking switches on and off until you locate the right one, so try not to overdo it. And don't forget smart lighting—dimmable bulbs controlled by remote-control devices or by an app on your smartphone—which allows you to tailor your lighting to morning or evening or to tasks. They are wireless, so they are tidy and can all be controlled from the one place; so if you're in the office you can switch your lights on with your mobile phone, and if you are going on holiday, no more setting a timer—you can simply set your lighting from your phone.

And if all this information sounds overwhelming, remember, many lighting suppliers will be happy to help you with your lighting plan.

LIGHTING TRICKS AND TIPS

So, lighting plan in hand, you're all set to discuss it with your architect (if you're really lucky) or, like many of us, you'll be making a trip to the lighting store. What else do you need to know before you set out?

- An uplighter in the corner of a room will bounce light upward and make the room look bigger.
- A ceiling-hung pendant lamp will make a room look taller.
- Lights under your wall-mounted kitchen cupboards will allow you to chop and cook without a shadow.
- A swivel lamp is perfect for reading or close work, but make sure that the lamp is tall enough

to be maneuverable, so there won't be shadows on the work.

- For bedside reading, make sure your lamp is adjustable—you don't want to have to crane your neck or assume an awkward position to relax and read!

- Clip-on lights are handy, as they can be moved around.

- You can use spotlights to highlight the things that you love, and integrated lighting in your wardrobe or hall cupboard to make things much easier to find. If integrated lighting is too expensive, LED spotlights can be cheaply installed; make sure you know what you are doing when installing lighting, though—if in doubt, contact an expert.

- Floor-level lighting is a good choice in areas like stairs and landings, where you don't want or need harsh lighting, particularly at night. Try LED strip lighting (see overleaf).

- When placing task lighting, if you are right-handed, place it to the left, or your hand will cast a shadow, and vice versa.

- Two lighting techniques—wall washing and light grazing—can add texture and a lovely sheen to a wall. A *wall washer* light is placed at a distance of more than 20cm (about eight inches) from the wall you want to highlight; with *light grazing* the light fitting is much closer, which can draw attention to the texture of a wall because of the angle of the light.

- LED strip lights are a really easy way to add light to task areas, such as the undersides of kitchen cupboards. These can be flexible and able to be installed anywhere, or more rigid and thus, of course, more durable, enabling them to be placed behind a picture or TV to provide interest. You can also place LED strip lights under your bathroom cabinet so that nighttime visits to the bathroom are not interrupted by harsh lighting.

- In the bedroom, choose a central light fitting that is restful, not too brightly colored or garish. Make sure it's dimmable and preferably with a remote control, so you won't have to get out of bed to turn the light off!

Lighting technicalities

As well as the practicalities, you'll need to acquaint yourself with some technical terms, and here we return to our old friends: lux and lumens, color temperature and the color rendering index (CRI). To recap: *Lux* is the measurement of light intensity, while *lumens* refers to the total amount of light that comes from a light source. One lux is equal to one lumen per square meter. If this sounds like Einstein's theory of relativity to you, basically, the more lumens, the brighter the light. Then, if you factor in the distance your light has to travel, you'll understand that the light from a central source might not fall as strongly on your newspaper as, say, that which comes from your desk lamp, because it has to travel farther. Another term that you might hear is *candela*, which is the unit of light intensity, with one candela being as bright as the light from one candle. As an example, a 60-watt bulb will provide 50 candelas of light—i.e., it'll be as bright as if you had lit 50 candles!

Here are some examples of the strength of light you'll need in the home:

- 100 lux in a living room

- 150 lux in a hallway

- 300 lux in a study

- 100 lux in a kitchen, but 300–400 at your countertop

- 50–100 lux in a bathroom, but 300–400 at your bathroom mirror

- 500 lux at a workbench in your garage

- 1,000 lux for precision work

The other thing to bear in mind is that the older we are, the stronger the light will need to be: A sixty-year-old will need three times more light than a twenty-year-old to do the same job.

Understanding color temperature

You may have heard light bulbs being described as "warm" or "cool." This doesn't refer to the temperature of the lamp itself but to its color, as we learned when we spoke about a filament being heated, and how its color would change from orange to yellow to bluish white as it got hotter (see page 40). So imagine a scale from 1,000K (very red) to 10,000K (very blue). It might seem counterintuitive when you think of a filament being heated, but *the higher up the scale you go, the closer the light resembles blue-white skylight.*

Why might you be interested in color temperature? Quite simply, it will set the mood of your space. Cool light promotes focus and precision work but is harsh on the complexion, whereas warm light is more hospitable and flattering. You can combine both types in the same room—for example, in a kitchen you may prefer a cool white lamp for work surfaces, but a warm white one above the dining table where people will gather. The food will look more appealing and your guests' faces more beautiful! The next time you buy a light bulb for your home, remember to check whether it is warm or cool—it will make all the difference. The Kelvin color temperature will be given on the bulb packaging, and often there will be a description on the front of the light output as "warm white" or "cool blue," and so on.

- Less than 3,300K is seen as warm light.

- 3,300–5,300K is experienced as neutral light.

- Higher than 5,300K is seen as cold light.

So if you'd like more warmth in your home, you'll know that candlelight has a lovely soft warmth to it, but so do the new vintage-look filament lamps, and a look at the packaging will tell you that their color temperature is 1,850K—i.e., ultra-warm. A standard incandescent is "warm" at 2,500K; a halogen incandescent, 3,000K, still warm; but a fluorescent tube is "cool," at 3,000–5,000K; and compact fluorescents and LEDs come in at 4,000K—very cool, as you can imagine, so you won't want to light your room fully with them!

Cool light promotes focus and precision work but is harsh on the complexion, whereas warm light is more hospitable and flattering.

Choosing your lights

When it comes to choosing lighting, you need to refer to the
CRI. This is a measure of how faithfully a light source reveals
the color of an object in comparison with the daylight standard.
You'll remember that the CRI is a scale from 0 to 100, indicating how accurately your eyes can detect subtle variations of color
under a given light source (see page 41). This has nothing to do
with the lamp's color temperature: You can have two lamps with
color temperatures of 2,800K, but how you see colors depends
on the CRI of each lamp.

Now, this might not seem important to you, but as humans
we need to see color accurately, and our brain health depends on
good-quality lighting with a high CRI. So check the CRI values
of any light bulbs you are buying—the information may not be
on the box, so you may have to ask the supplier. Use the table
below as a guide.

100 is absolutely perfect Sunlight and certain
fine incandescent bulbs such as halogen attain this
value. Interestingly, the humble incandescent bulb
has this value, so it may well have its uses, as modern
replacements haven't been able to match its CRI.
Interestingly, when the US government initiated a
competition to design a low-energy light bulb with a
high CRI, the winner, a 60W LED light bulb with a
CRI of 93, did not attain commercial traction, probably
due to expense.[55]

90 gives minimal color distortions LED lights tend to
operate at around 80–90—the lowest value for healthy
color rendering.

80 gives small color distortions Fluorescent discharge tubes often only measure 80.

70 is the minimum for color vision and only to be used for secondary areas Cheaper versions of fluorescents drop to a CRI of 70. These systematically feed the eyes incorrect chromatic information.

The parameters of color rendering are defined by the International Commission on Illumination (CIE), and the standard is currently being upgraded and expanded. Keep an eye out for new types of technical data and ask your lighting supplier to explain them.

If your room is on the gloomy side, try a soft pastel shade, which will add warmth and brighten the space. The rule of thumb is, if you have to turn the light on during the day, white is not the color for you.

Using color wisely

It's also important to consider your color scheme when you are trying to maximize light in the home. It's no accident that my fellow Swedes favor pale, light colors in interior design. But don't be fooled into painting a gloomy space white to light it—sometimes this can make it look grubby; white, ironically, often looks best in an already-bright space, where the sunlight bounces off it. If your room is on the gloomy side, try a soft pastel shade, which will add warmth and brighten the space. The rule of thumb is, if you have to turn the light on during the day, white is not the color for you. Try a peach, a warm beige, or a soft dove gray. Buy samples of paint and try them in your room—paint a nice big patch to get a proper idea. And paint your samples onto different walls so that you can judge the different light settings. Finally, it may sound counterintuitive, but sometimes the only way to deal with a dark space is to embrace it and paint it a muted color so that it becomes a cozy nook—a nest, if you like.

MAGIC WITH MIRRORS

Mirrors are an excellent way of brightening up spaces. You can be adventurous here: For special effects, glass crystals and plastic prisms will cast beautiful colored rainbows on surrounding walls.

For internal use:

- Place a mirror opposite a window to reflect light and any outdoor greenery.

- A cluster of small mirrors of different shapes creates interesting light patterns in gloomy corners.

- Turning a long rectangular mirror on its side will make a short wall look longer and create an interesting reflection of your room. A long vertical mirror will make your ceiling feel higher.

- Place a mirror behind a light source for pretty reflections.

You can also use mirrors outdoors, and thus add a whole new dimension to a plant-filled corner. Or try sheets of polished stainless steel—they won't rust and are safe around children. Sheets of shiny stainless steel can be found at wholesale metal suppliers; have them cut to size, and fix them on windowsills and facing facades.

USING COLORED LIGHT IN THE HOME

In a home setting, we think of "color" in terms of interior decorating—paint, furnishings, and fabrics—but what about colored light? By this, I don't mean what we've been talking about regarding "warm" and "cool" light and CRIs; I mean actual colored light. Why not? If you think about it, we are surrounded by the reflected light of different colors bouncing off fabric, wallpaper, or paint, but their luminous intensity is quite low. The colored light coming directly from a lamp is much stronger and has a pronounced biological impact. A general rule is to add energizing light colors to promote activity, and soothing hues to encourage calm, so bluish-white light will make us feel alert and concentrated in an office or study, for example, but the direction of the incoming light is important. Bluish radiation must always come from a large surface overhead. Our old biological habits want the luminous heavens to be high above us—so fit bluish-white lights above your work space.

However, do not use bluish lights late at night: In a study for the *Journal of Neuroscience* in 2013 on Siberian hamsters, it was found that exposure to blue light produced adverse effects on their brains and, in short, more depressive symptoms. By contrast, the little creatures seemed much happier with red light, and the authors of the study, Professor Randy Nelson and Dr.

Tracy Bedrosian, came to the conclusion that "the findings may have important implications for humans, particularly those whose work on night shifts makes them susceptible to mood disorders. . . . Our findings suggest that if we could use red light when appropriate for night-shift workers, it may not have some of the negative effects on their health that white light does."

So if we follow the hamster example, red light is excellent at night. Once you have gone to sleep, your body gets to work on internal regenerative processes and should not be disturbed. But what if you need to get up in the middle of the night to visit the toilet or perhaps the fridge? Switching on a bright white light will shock your system into daytime mode and disrupt your sleep. Try fitting a red light to your bathroom for those night-time visits. Many modern lighting systems—the "smart" ones that can be controlled by an app—will also provide color lighting, so the world is your oyster, but respect your old rhythms, because they are there for a reason: to safeguard your physical and mental well-being.

For a million years, evening meals have been served by golden firelight, so it comes as no surprise that this color range is well suited for kitchens or dining rooms. Moreover, orange light is cosmetically very flattering to the human skin—your dinner guests will look great and social interaction will be much enhanced. Why not also introduce a touch of orange light into bathrooms and bedrooms? These are places we spend time looking in the mirror—if we look good, we feel good. The bedroom in particular is a good place to use orange light. Our brains have been conditioned to respond to this color cue and start producing the sleep hormone melatonin, so feed yourself small doses of soft orange light before bedtime, ideally from a low-level light source that "washes" the floor with an amber glow. This is how early humans experienced firelight for cooking and protection. If this seems too much trouble, simply buy a low-wattage, soft orange light bulb and fit it to your bedside lamp. Some of these are even marketed as sleep-enhancing. Alternatively, using an orange lampshade is the easiest way to achieve an amber ambience.

Deep green has a psychologically soothing and calming effect while still promoting focus. Indeed, reading is best done against a green background—who doesn't love the restful green lamps in an old library? But green light is rarely used for household purposes, as it is not pretty on the human face—none of us looks good in green light! Nonetheless, accents of green light are a delight in a sitting room, as green illumination will supply the body clock with the much-needed middle portion of the visible spectrum. (The normal eye has its highest sensitivity in mid-spectrum at 555nm.) As we'll recall, green is the color of the African forest, where human sight originated.

And finally, a word about the new innovation that is dynamic lighting systems. These exciting new systems try to imitate the color of the solar phases during the day. LED technology has made the automatic color tuning of the different lamps relatively easy. They are mostly programmed for cool bluish light in the morning hours to awaken the brain. Luminous levels will peak around noon when your body expects a high rate of activity. Toward afternoon and evening, a reddish hue resembling sunset kicks in. Physiological functions start to wind down and the body prepares itself for the quiet of the evening.

Dynamic lighting is expensive, so it hasn't reached private homes yet, but it is beginning to be used more in institutions and offices, as we realize the benefits of replicating natural light in indoor spaces. One interesting study, conducted by the Korean Institute for Advanced Technology, compared lighting effects on students in two math classes, one of which was using the "standard" fluorescent lighting, and the other of which was treated to LED lights. The results were an improvement in the "LED" students' math scores, and also in their feeling of well-being.

Dynamic lighting is gaining ground in the educational sector; however, it is sometimes an inexact science, as natural light varies a lot more throughout the day than artificial light, and the gradations from dawn to dusk can be dramatic. The technology of these systems is not advanced enough to factor in such finely tuned variations—we still need to spend quality time outdoors to maximize the biological benefits of natural daylight.

Which brings me back to the beginning of this chapter. As human beings, we are now beginning to understand the importance of spending more time outdoors, and also of modifying our relationship with electric light, so long considered a boon to humanity. We are now turning our attention to its effects on both animals and humans—indeed, on the future of our industrialized society. We are doing this at a time of enormous technological change, which has great benefits in terms of new developments such as human-centric and smart lighting, and which can help us to raise awareness of the impact of electric lighting in our lives. Electric light can do fantastic things in our homes, now more than ever, with the advent of LEDs, but the price can be high in terms of our age-old circadian rhythms. It's clear to me that we'll need to find another way forward as we progress into the twenty-first century, in which work and technological advances are balanced with a new respect for nature and for natural light.

THE LIGHT DIET

Let food be thy medicine and medicine be thy food.

—HIPPOCRATES

In this chapter, I'll look at how you can maximize your health and well-being by following a sensible, healthy "light" diet. When I say eating a healthy "light" diet, I mean a diet that nourishes the body's five light "gateways": the eyes, brain, blood, skin, and ligaments. Let's see how to assist them by feeding them nourishing, tasty food and by keeping irritants to a minimum.

Nowadays, we are increasingly aware of the role of healthy eating in our lives, and of how processed foods can negatively impact our well-being. Recent data shows that, particularly in northern countries, we are eating a great deal of processed food, with shopping baskets in some countries containing up to 50 percent "ultra-processed food," i.e., food that is high in saturated fat, refined carbohydrate, salt, and additives. In this we differ strikingly from our southern European neighbors. In

Portugal, for example, a shopping basket will contain only 10 percent of these unhealthy foods.[56] Of course, the purpose of this chapter is not to deliver a lecture, but to act as a reminder that what we eat affects who we are, and that in the fight against diseases such as diabetes, we all have a part to play. By eating wholesome "real" food, we are treating not only our bodies, but also our senses.

Many fresh foods that we buy have been grown with the use of pesticides. A simple wash with water and a tiny drop of liquid soap will help to remove residues, but if you are concerned by this, you can, of course, choose organic food—although it is expensive and not in everyone's budget. If you would like to take a closer look at pesticides in food, the European Food Safety Authority provides data on pesticide residues in European countries and in a number of different fruits and vegetables.[57] As a rule of thumb, look for vegetables and fruit that have been naturally grown under plentiful sun and haven't been forced in any way—consuming them is an indirect way of eating photonic energy. Local produce is best, but realistically, your climate zone may not supply this throughout the year—just do your best to eat local whenever you can: It makes sense that the less distance the food has had to travel, the fresher it will be.

FOODS FOR THE EYES AND BRAIN

The functioning of the eye–brain system is intimately influenced by the functioning of the digestive tract, but, more to the point, if we eat a healthy diet, we will help to combat many of the eye problems that are linked to diseases such as diabetes and heart disease.

Chard, spinach, broccoli, kale, and green peppers

Eat plenty of dark green leafy vegetables that are naturally saturated with the light-harvesting molecule chlorophyll. Under the influence of strong sunlight this is transformed into the coenzyme quinone, which activates the mitochondria inside every cell in your body. These tiny energy reactors will power your entire body. Spinach is cheap and abundant and an excellent source of lutein, which can protect cells from damage.

Pumpkins, carrots, beets, tomatoes, and berries

Orange and red vegetables contain large amounts of organic pigments also known as "bioflavonoids." These concentrated carotene colorants also act as efficient antioxidants, which are thought to help in eye, skin, and heart health. Beta-carotene, which is found in yellow and orange fruits and vegetables, is converted to vitamin A in the body, excellent for heart and eye health.

Avocados, walnuts, coconuts, olives, and organic butter

While the health benefits of avocados, walnuts, and coconuts have now been embraced, people are still hesitant about butter. This might be because until quite recently all health advice suggested that "fat" was bad for us. We now know that this message has been oversimplified and, more to the point, that so-called "diet" foods replaced saturated fat with unhealthy sugars and additives. We understand that we need certain "good" fats for our health. These saturated and semi-saturated fat sources are all of natural origin. They have an excellent balance between their omega-3 and omega-6 components. Butter contains vitamin A and is one of the most complex of all dietary fats, containing more than four hundred fatty acids. All body cells are enclosed in double layers of fatty membranes, and these elastic wrappings must be well nourished to fulfill their function. Brain tissue is particularly high in fat since the nerve cells are externally lined with lipid cells, acting as efficient electric insulators. Yes, butter is saturated but contains butyric acid, which is important for the digestive enzymes. Organic butter is a natural product that undergoes minimal processing in contrast to industrial oils.

Yogurt, cheese, eggs, soybeans, and seafood

These proteins are complete and contain all the essential amino acids that your body needs. High-grade proteins are easily converted into functional tissue. An extra supply is vital to recycle and repair the discarded old membranes inside the retinal cells. The brain also needs a lot of prime-quality proteins to build trillions of internal nerve connections.

Eyebright, dandelion, rosehips, green tea, fennel, saffron, turmeric, chili, and garlic

These organic tonics will fortify and cleanse your inner organs and tissues but won't overstimulate your body. Many wild herbs and spices improve blood circulation and strengthen the immune system. Most are slightly bitter in taste but high in vitamins and natural antibiotics. Some are antibacterial and full of yellow antioxidant pigments.

FOODS RICH IN EYE- AND BRAIN-NOURISHING VITAMINS AND MINERALS

The eye and brain cells use up a tremendous amount of energy and need powerful antioxidants to protect the mitochondria. The mitochondria are the energy processors in our cells, which take in nutrients and break them down in a process known as "cellular respiration." Again, it's a complex process, but when we think about it, a miraculous one: to consider that everything we eat is providing our body with nutrients at a cellular level. Of course, this means that we need to ensure that we are getting the vitamins we need, and ideally from natural sources: You can take large doses of vitamin C and your body will simply dispose of what it doesn't need, but on the other hand, large doses of vitamin A and vitamin D can be toxic. As in everything, the key is balance. Dark green, leafy vegetables and brightly colored vegetables are good sources of vitamin A; citrus fruit will supply you with plentiful vitamin C; and many cereals and milks are fortified with vitamin B12, which is also available in cheese, eggs, and seafood. Vitamin E can be found in sunflower seeds, almonds, hazelnuts, oily fish, and some seafood, such as lobster. And if lobster is out of your price range, try trout, or cheaper vegetables such as sweet potatoes or butternut squash—or even olive oil. But please consider how you cook and serve your vegetables. Avoid overcooking them, thereby causing them to lose valuable nutrients.

For optimum functioning of your eyes, you'll also need certain essential minerals and trace elements, including calcium, magnesium, selenium, and zinc. These affect capillary blood flow and nerve conduction, and influence the contraction of the fine-control muscles. As with all vitamins and minerals, try to get them from the food you eat rather than taking concentrated supplements. Nuts are a very good source of a range of minerals, as are beans, lentils, and leafy greens. If you are a meat eater, you are in luck, as beef contains a number of minerals, as do fish and shellfish. If you don't eat meat, tofu contains calcium, which is good news for vegans, in addition to minerals such as phosphorus and iron. Calcium can, of course, be found in dairy products such as milk, yogurt, and cheese, but it's also in leafy greens such as kale and bok choy, as well as fortified "plant" milks—check before you buy your favorite milk that it is fortified with calcium. It will be marked on the carton.

IRRITANTS TO THE EYES AND BRAIN

We've looked at delicious healthy foods to optimize eye and brain function, but we must be equally aware of irritants. These include concentrated and industrially refined foods or even food substitutes, which may be connected to the process of producing "free radicals." Free radicals have been implicated in a number of human diseases due to "oxidative stress," in which proteins, lipids, and DNA are altered. The body's natural defenses are not equipped to handle this sudden flare-up and, among other things, the delicate cellular membranes of the eyes will become damaged. Many studies have pointed to the role of oxidative stress in "dry eye" disease, among others,[58] and it pays to limit our consumption of these foodstuffs. Margarine is highly processed, but certain polyunsaturated oils can also react with light.[59] Free radicals are released when polyunsaturated fats oxidize under strong light.[60]

Refined white flour

Intensive milling and processing have removed all fibers, minerals, and vitamins from the natural grain. White flour is high in starch and gluten that clog up the digestive system and cause allergies in some people. Constipation is also a factor to consider with overconsumption of refined flour products.

Coffee, tea, cola, chocolate, and tobacco

Attractive though they may be, these products contain naturally occurring alkaloids, chemical compounds that have been used in many drugs, from opium to antidepressants. The ancient Egyptians were known to use alkaloid-containing plants for their psychotropic properties, as indeed were native South Americans with their "coca" leaves. However, as you can imagine, these are powerful stimulants that stress the nervous system and as a consequence disrupt your sleep. Many alkaloid-containing plants and substances do have some nutritional value, but tend to raise blood pressure, so consume in strict moderation, and when it comes to tobacco, the ideal is not at all.

Refined white sugar

You'll probably have heard quite a lot of discussion recently about the role of sugar in our diets. Now we are told that all sugar is "bad" for us, even the naturally occurring sugars we find in fruit. However, while it's true to say that our body processes sugar as sugar, fruit also provides us with fiber, vitamins, and minerals. On the other hand, white sugar is a nonfood from which all nutrients have been removed. It is a powerful stimulant that burns the delicate linings of your blood vessels and depletes the body's stores of chromium. A much-researched sugar-related symptom is diabetes, a disease that has ultimately been shown to damage the eyesight.

For many of us, the problem with sugar is overconsumption. The World Health Organization (WHO) recommends consumption of no more than six teaspoons of sugar a day. However, when you consider that the average fizzy drink contains seven teaspoons of sugar, and a tin of baked beans contains four teaspoons of sugar, it's easy to see how it can all add up. *Added* sugar is the culprit here—i.e., sugar that has been added to our food artificially. Try to cut down on foods without naturally occurring sugars. Of course, you might well wonder how you can do this, when so much sugar is hidden in our food, but getting label-wise is the key. A look through the ingredients list will help; some foods will be high in naturally occurring sugars, so you won't necessarily be able to tell, but if "sugar" is near the top of the list, you'll know that the product contains a lot of it. If you see the words "glucose" or "fructose syrup" or "rice malt syrup," you will be eating sugar, and of a particularly potent kind.

And a note about sugars such as honey, agave syrup, and molasses. They may taste nice and you may think that they are better for you, but they are still sugar, and your body will process them in the same way, so don't be tempted to substitute these for your teaspoon of sugar in coffee—and then eat a slice of cheesecake to boot! Reduce your overall (added) sugar intake by replacing sugary foods with foods high in natural fats and protein to fill you up for longer and keep the sugar cravings at bay.[61]

MSG (monosodium glutamate)

This chemical is used in some cuisines as a flavor enhancer and has been linked by some consumers to a range of symptoms including sweating, numbness in certain areas, and chest pain. The US Food and Drug Administration (FDA) has declared the food "safe," but as many report anecdotal symptoms, such as headaches, it is required to be listed as part of an ingredients list.

FOODS FOR THE SKIN

The skin is the outer envelope that protects and nurtures your body—think of it as an organic space suit with a remarkable capacity for self-repair. Of course, it is not as light-sensitive as the eyes, but compensates because of the sheer volume of its fine capillary mesh. Before you expose your beautiful skin to full radiant sunlight—and we have discussed the benefits and the dangers in chapter 3—bolster its natural strength and resilience with good nutrition.

Sweet almonds and macadamia nuts

These tasty nuts and their oils will never oxidize or go rancid. They don't spontaneously decay and are thus used in costly cosmetic creams. Eating them is, of course, a much more efficient way of benefiting from their nutrition.

Yogurt

After sun exposure, yogurt is a great coolant for the digestive system. It's no accident that Indian cuisine has many yogurt-based drinks to counteract the spices in the food. The high content of lactic acid and probiotics also helps the friendly bacteria in your gut to multiply. Applying it to your skin can help with sunburn, although you might prefer aloe vera!

MELANIN BOOSTERS

According to the University of Maryland, tyrosine "is an essential component for the production of several important brain chemicals, called neurotransmitters." Additionally, melanin is a "polymer"—a chain of molecules—of tyrosine and, as we know, melanin is the brown pigment layer generated by our skin as UV protection. We need melanin, so eating tyrosine-containing foods will help to boost our production of that pigment. It's naturally found in turkey, Parmesan cheese, avocados, and almonds.

IRRITANTS TO THE SKIN

Feeding and looking after your skin properly will do much to keep its defenses strong. But some plants and foods irritate the skin and react negatively in combination with strong sunlight. This effect is known as "phototoxicity." You will notice the following list includes some natural, health-promoting foods, and this doesn't mean you should never use them. It really depends on where you are in the world, and the season.

Dill, mustard, ginger, vanilla, and citrus oils

Aromatic plants that contain concentrated essential oils can act as powerful skin irritants. The allergenic effect is enhanced when you are exposed to strong light. Perhaps you've spilled orange or lime juice on a T-shirt while out in the sun and your skin has blistered? That's phototoxicity.

Buckwheat

Tasty and nutritious it may be, but buckwheat contains fagopyrin, which can cause phototoxicity. For us humans, eating the seeds or using buckwheat flour is generally considered to be fine, but animals eating a lot of these plants have been found to develop skin rashes and eye ulcers when grazing under strong sunlight, so while we might not suffer if we eat buckwheat, it's wise not to overdo consumption.

CHEMICAL CARE

Food is not the only contributor to phototoxicity. Photo-allergenic chemicals may be natural or man-made and can be found in things like medicines, solvents, perfumes, and—paradoxically—artificial sunscreens. Ultraviolet light changes the structure of these chemicals and they are attacked by the immune system. Autoimmune reactions damage body tissue. Read the labels of products carefully before you use them in the sun. The following table will help you identify some of the main photo-allergenic chemicals to avoid.

- Sulfa—used in some drugs, among them some antibiotics, diuretics, COX-2 inhibitors, and diabetes drugs

- Psoralens, coal tars, photoactive dyes (eosin, acridine orange)
- Musk ambrette, methylcoumarin, lemon oil (may be present in fragrances)
- PABA (found in sunscreens)
- Oxybenzone (UVA and UVB chemical blocker in sunscreens)
- Salicylanilide (found in industrial cleaners)
- St. John's wort (used to treat depression)
- Hexachlorophene (found in some antibacterial soaps)
- Contact with sap from giant hogweed. Common rue is another phototoxic plant commonly found in gardens
- Tetracycline antibiotics

Everyone should avoid excessive sun exposure, but people who are sensitive to sunlight for any reason should be especially careful and wear protective clothes, avoid direct sunlight, and use sunscreens regularly. Talk to your doctor about alternatives to drugs that may cause photosensitivity, but if you are taking drugs with these side effects, heed your doctor's warning about their interactions with sunlight.

FOODS FOR THE PINEAL GLAND

We discussed the pineal gland earlier in the book (see page 60), but to recap, it's one of the master glands in the body, located in the middle of the brain. It is highly photosensitive and produces the sleep hormone melatonin that rules your diurnal rhythms. The pineal also has many other functions: It controls body temperature, sexual maturity, and the conversion of nerve signals. To function properly, the gland needs daily doses of strong daylight coupled with regular cycles of deep darkness. Taking substances such as caffeine, particularly late at night, alcohol, and sleeping pills will interfere with this finely balanced mechanism. Try not to overindulge. If you are taking sleeping tablets for whatever reason, try to take them for the shortest time possible to avoid disrupting your natural cycle.

FOODS FOR THE BLOOD

The blood is a dynamic oxygen carrier and its functioning is closely linked to healthy hemoglobin, which is the protein molecule in red blood cells. Hemoglobin helps the blood to transport much-needed oxygen to our tissues and to transport carbon monoxide back to be exhaled by the lungs. Easily absorbed iron is critical for the production of new red blood cells, and we need to eat iron-rich foods to ensure a good supply of this mineral. Many of the good food sources are themselves red-colored.

Beef, lamb, turkey, liver, and eggs

The sources that the body finds easiest to absorb come from animals and are known as "heme irons." It's important not to overdo iron consumption, however, as high levels of organic iron can cause constipation.

Shrimp, oysters, and sardines

Fish and seafood also contain rich amounts of iron of the valuable heme type.

Spinach, parsley, lentils, broccoli, red chilis, tomatoes, strawberries, raisins, and molasses

Non-heme irons are found in many vegetable sources, although they aren't as readily absorbed as the first group. To improve uptake, combine them with foods naturally rich in vitamin C, or include a little animal protein in the meal. If you are a vegetarian, talk to your doctor about taking supplements—a blood test can be done to gauge amounts and determine whether a supplement is needed.

Herring, salmon, avocados, walnuts, and flaxseed

Your blood also contains small repair cells called platelets, which can cause clotting and restrict the blood's natural flow. Some foods have a blood-thinning effect and will improve general circulation. All the foods listed above contain vital omega-3 fatty acids.

IRRITANTS TO THE BLOOD

If you don't have enough healthy red blood cells, you may ultimately suffer from iron-deficiency anemia. It is more common among women than men, as women lose blood during their menstrual periods and may also experience low iron levels during pregnancy and breastfeeding. Finding a good source of iron isn't as easy for vegetarians and vegans as it is for meat eaters, particularly if you omit cheese, eggs, and milk from your diet. If you do follow a vegan diet—and it's a popular choice nowadays—consult a nutritionist to make sure that you are getting the right amount of vitamins and minerals in your diet.

External threats to your hemoglobin levels may come from the environment. We know that hemoglobin binds with both oxygen and carbon monoxide, but the monoxide forms a chemical bond that is eight times stronger. Once in place, it blocks access to any other molecule, including vital oxygen. Your primary sources of this toxic carbon gas are tobacco smoke, car fumes, and candles. Yes, candles! A few tea lights in a well-ventilated room or a couple of candles over dinner won't cause problems, but don't burn lots of candles at once, particularly in a room that isn't well ventilated.

And finally, there is more to blood health than eating a lot of good iron for hemoglobin. The enriched blood has to circulate to transport oxygen and remove all toxic waste products. Do some physical exercise to improve the flow of blood and lymph and to make yourself feel better. There is no better natural pick-me-up than exercise, ideally outdoors on a lovely light-filled day.

LIGHT THROUGHOUT YOUR LIFE

A healthy, light diet will certainly help us to optimize our light consumption, but it also helps to be aware of how we respond to light throughout the course of our lives, whether we are male or female, old or young, "larks" or "owls." When we are teenagers, for example, hormonal changes affect our body clocks (which those of us with teenage children will no doubt have witnessed), and so we go to sleep later and wake up later. It can be a real struggle for teens to get out of bed on school mornings. The answer is to get them out during the daytime more. It might also be good to consider buying them a dawn simulator, which will wake them up gradually.

Light for old age

When we age, we find that we sleep less, and this is because the pineal gland in the brain shrinks with age, meaning that the natural production of the sleep hormone melatonin decreases. Little babies can slumber around the clock, while the elderly experience shortened periods of sleep. Bright light in the afternoon will encourage a shift toward a more delayed cycle. Also, try to limit alcohol and caffeine, both favorites with older people. They are irritants to the pineal gland and won't help you sleep.

If you are older, you might also have noticed that colors seem less vivid. This is because the eye's lens is hardening, and its transparent protein crystals are changing from yellow to brown. Thus, for senior eyes, yellow objects will stand out in their full glory, while blue objects will appear grayish and dull. Yellow is therefore a good visual marker for where extra attention is needed, and color contrast will also help. Try to avoid monotone white in the bathroom, for example, to minimize the risk of slipping.

Older people might also benefit from light therapy, and a light box switched on while you are eating your breakfast or reading your newspaper will make you feel brighter and may well improve your nighttime sleep. Finally, older bodies have more difficulty in converting solar energy into vitamin D, so sunbathing *with care* can help to replenish your stocks of this important vitamin. Culturally, you might feel awkward exposing your skin, but vitamin D is vital for aging bodies.

Light for men and women

We may not like to admit it, but there are differences in the way men and women see. Neuroscience has confirmed it! Women's color vision is better than men's, as the psychologist Dr. Israel Abramov of the City University of New York has discovered. In a series of tests administered to volunteers, he found that women could spot more subtle variations in color, whereas men fared better in tests involving distant moving objects. The reasons are biological, and possibly evolutionary, as men were originally hunter-gatherers and needed to see farther.[62] However, as to why more men than women are color-blind, it is thought to be genetic, with 8 percent of men (of northern European ancestry) being color-blind as opposed to 0.5 percent of women.[63] Interestingly, indigenous people, both men and women, in tropical and Arctic regions exhibit no color-vision deficiency at all.

Sadly, SAD is more prevalent among women. Be aware of the symptoms of SAD. If you find yourself battling fatigue and the blues during the winter months, find ways of increasing your consumption of daylight. Try to get outside at lunchtime if you can. You might also find a light box helpful—but choose carefully, as there are many on the market. Monochromatic light therapy can also help, if it is available in your area, for a color boost.

Light for night vision

Night blindness is something that can trouble us increasingly as we get older, for a number of reasons: our irises grow weaker and our pupils shrink—according to Harvard Health, this can be by as much as 2mm. Consequently, our pupils can take longer to adjust to dimmer lighting, or can struggle when going from a brightly lit environment to a dimly lit one. A cloudy lens can also be a culprit, as can the decline in the number and functioning of rods in the eye.[64] There is some research to suggest that vitamin A plays a part in alleviating night-vision problems, particularly for those in the developing world. Eating vitamin-A-rich foods, such as carrots, sweet potatoes, and kale, can help, of course, but there is also a school of thought that suggests that increasing cholesterol interferes with vitamin A absorption, so eat a healthy, balanced diet, with lots of plants in it—and pay attention to your light habits.

Light for fertility

If you are thinking of starting a family, it might interest you to know that bright morning light may have a positive effect on reproductive hormone stimulation, and may also help to correct irregular periods. Artificial light also has some therapeutic benefits. Japanese research has shown that women can irradiate face and breast areas with red light to stimulate milk production.[65]

If you find the above a little far-fetched, many experimental examples show that external light intake has a fundamental influence on animal and human fertility. Among Eskimo women at extreme Arctic latitudes, for example, menstrual periods come to a full halt during the darkest months of winter, and regular ovulation does not resume until the reappearance of solar light. By contrast, women of the tropics are fully fertile all year-round, despite malnutrition and starvation.

Midwives know that twice as many babies are born in spring compared to autumn—implying that the infants were conceived around the summer solstice when the light levels are at a maximum. Male sexuality is likewise strongly enhanced during the brightest months of the year. Sunshine stimulates the testes to forceful growth with abundant production of vigorous sperm.

Part of the experimental knowledge we have gleaned is regularly and ruthlessly employed in animal breeding. A healthy hen will normally lay an egg per day, but this can be manipulated by doubling the light cycles during the same time span. With electrical dimmers, two sunrises and sunsets can be imitated at an accelerated tempo. The poor bird thinks that two days have elapsed in the span of twenty-four hours and does her best not to lose track of her solar reproductive cycle.

Chinchillas kept under red illumination during conception and gestation will give birth to an excess of male pups. Blue light will give a surplus of young females with softer fur than the males, who are thus commercially more valuable. Similar experiments have also been performed on mice. When kept in blue light during the pregnancy phase, they bore about 70 percent female pups in the litter, while irradiation with red gave the opposite outcome.

Twin births is another area that also proves to be light dependent. In the equatorial area, identical twins are so extraordinarily rare that they are given semi-divine status. But the farther north or south one travels, the more frequent twins become. In the harsh tundra in the extreme north of Finland, all fecundity records are broken with the world's highest rate of twin births.

It seems appropriate that I end this journey through light with the stages of life, because this wonder that we take so much for granted is with us from birth to old age; it marks the beginning of each day and the fading of the light marks its end. It's an age-old ritual that rules all of life on earth. In fact, we are now becoming increasingly aware of the costs of ignoring this ritual as progress pulls us on. I find it fascinating—and reassuring—to understand just how important light is to life and to know that, rather than dismissing it in our twenty-four-hour lifestyles, we can harness it, learn more about it, and use it to live better, happier lives. I hope that this book has given you insights into this wonder, and that it has also helped you in practical ways to bring more light into your life.

When I first opened Monocrom in Stockholm all those years ago, my aims were simple: to provide solace to my fellow Swedes who were suffering during our long, dark winters. I quickly realized that this was only the beginning of my life's work, to understand more about the magic of light and to share it with you. In *Living Light*, I hope that I have been able to do this and, more important, that you have enjoyed taking this journey through light with me.

APPENDIX

THE COLOR GALLERY

Color is an essential part of our lives. Millions of years ago, humans would have had limited color vision; however, we have evolved to see all the colors of a rainbow, as indeed have chimps and gorillas.

A million years ago, the domestication of fire and use of simple tools sharpened the human senses, enhancing precision and discrimination, so keen vision became more important. The ordering of the primary colors in opposing pairs—red/green and blue/yellow, for example—offered practical advantages. In outdoor life, contrary, or complementary, colors would often indicate contrasting phenomena of great importance: water versus fire or night versus day.

The four ancients

Red

The most significant color of the primitive quadruple of four colors is unquestionably red. Ancient archaeological pigment findings are all based on reddish ocher. The color sensation is intimately connected with the spilling of blood, and most primates become nervous when they see it. The human eye detects red objects faster than anything else, and it is usually the first color name a child will utter. Objects in strong reds appear to be closer and larger than in real life. They stimulate the sympathetic nervous system to increase pulse rate and body temperature. Intensely warm tones of red can invigorate body strength, particularly in cases of fatigue or muscle recovery, excellent for a gym or physiotherapy room. Passionate reds also boost both sexuality and self-confidence. Heavy doses can be distinctly stress-inducing, however, and raging red is contraindicative in cases of anger or impatience. Avoid using red in environments where people are accident-prone or aggressive. You have never seen a police officer in a red uniform!

Green

Most terrestrial animals associate green with fertile pastures offering protection, food, and water. Lush foliage would have given us shelter from predators, and even modern flocks of stressed humans find green soothing. Green is well suited to therapeutic settings and gives a friendly, emotional touch. This color connects to deep-seated biological memories and is pleasantly neutral beyond warm or cold. Green is eye-catching, and notably so if the vista is composed of living plants.

Our past, which would have originally been spent in verdant jungles, means that our vision has adapted to operate against a backdrop of green. In this color, our eyes will focus precisely, which is why you might find reading easiest against a green background—it's no accident that many chalkboards and reading desks in libraries were green.

Yellow

Our tropical ancient past means that bright tones of yellow are almost universally associated with sunshine in our brains. In sun-starved countries, during the dark winter months, many of us dream about the sun! Yellow is also biologically and emotionally linked to our daytime cycles. We are diurnal creatures, and the rising morning star means the start of an active day. Yellow is mentally activating and stimulates the brain, which is why it is the color of classrooms and venues for creative conferences or lively discussions. However, larger surfaces of sharp yellow can overstimulate, so it should be used sparingly, as symptoms of migraine or vertigo are easily aggravated. That is why yellow is never used in airplane cabins. Older people have enhanced visual perception of this color, and clear golden highlights will help them navigate; yellow on a handrail will help prevent an elderly person from stumbling.

Blue

Modern humans love blue! It is linked to the night cycle and chronobiologically heralds dusk and twilight, turning into midnight blue. When we look at blue, our pupils contract, and blue objects seem more distant. Deep blue is an excellent relaxant and the perfect color for a bedroom or hotel room. The parasympathetic nervous system is activated by the color blue, and our pulse, blood pressure, and muscle tonus decrease, while our body temperature sinks and our breathing gets deeper. However, blue pigment isn't the same as blue light, which will stimulate us. By contrast, the *color* blue has great therapeutic value in cases of hypertension and insomnia, as it lulls us into a state of relaxation—which is why noisy and crowded venues benefit from generous doses of blue. However, a heavy dose of blue isn't good for those of us who have a tendency toward depression, as it can cause us to literally get "the blues."

The four newcomers

Orange

Early tribes would have gathered around the orange light of a fire as a collective symbol of safety, warmth, and cooking. This color is highly edible, and many of the foods we consume are in the gold-orange-brown range. Orange is cosmetically most flattering to the human skin: A golden-orange room will make your guests glow with a healthy radiance. Many cosmetic products are based on the orange palette.

Turquoise

The watery color of deep oceans and cool springs. Also known as aquamarine, it is refreshing and hygienic, a color perfectly suited for a washtub or a bathroom. Turquoise blinds will cool an office with windows facing the sun. Psychologically, it is a very sober color, and we associate it with privacy and aloofness.

Lime

The fresh color of early spring days with burgeoning leaves and electric-yellow-green buds. Emotionally, it has antidepressive effects, and after a long, gray winter, it can make people laugh again. Used for curtains, it will let a euphoric feeling of spring enter the room. It signals the start of new projects and wild plans.

Purple

A color we associate with late autumn, with flowering heather, ripening plums, and blushing grapes. The plant world heralds harvesttime and approaching death with a last glowing display of purple. Catholics use the color for mourning, and religious dignitaries have long favored it as an indicator of spiritual maturity. Purple is the color of departure and widowhood, when all is old and nature is about to close for the season. Human seniority may be accompanied with ripeness and possibly wisdom. Therapeutically, it speaks of emotional healing from lifelong experience. Purple rooms breathe solemnity, with a feeling of ritual.

The basic neutrals

Although they don't carry focal information, background tones provide us with useful contextual ideas of space, layout, and direction. Our natural scenery generously provides us with neutral shades of sand, stone, or wood, all nonintrusive and elegantly calming, but in the long run not very exciting!

Grays

In the neutral scale of white-gray-black we find the "achromatic," or colorless, tones. They are totally devoid of chromatic information but offer a faint backdrop that we tend to associate with the winter season: pebbles and stone, sleet and snow, gravel and bark. Grays are popular among designers and architects, as neutral and impersonal background notes. They are ideal for a textiles lab, where nothing must disrupt exact color judgment. However, as a visual "main course," they will eventually cause emotional fatigue due to their lack of stimulation.

Browns

The subdued tones of the earth link to our biological origins, and to farming as the original simple way of life. A sense of deep emotional protection can be drawn from the soil in rural environments. Browns were never glamorous or flashy, with poverty lurking just around the corner, but recent trends for costly coffee and exotic chocolate have made them quite fashionable. Browns and beiges also indicate organic products free from artificial colorants.

Metals

This is a special family of burnished colors reflecting light, like shiny metallic mirrors. Any color can be overlaid on a specular surface to obtain the familiar sheen of silver, gold, bronze, or copper, allowing new metallic shades to be produced, for example, in the range green-blue-purple. The latter lack established names (we have proper names for metallic red [copper] and orange [bronze] but not for metallic green or blue) but are much appreciated by both humans and animals. Insects, birds, and fish are immediately attracted to lustrous metallic surfaces and avidly select the glossiest partners available. The lure of glitter is irresistible, and magpies will, without guilt, snatch away your polished silver spoons. Even car-owning humans are enamored with the magic sheen of metals, and women love it for jewelry.

COLOR THERAPY

But what about colors as therapeutic agents? Surely color is more than just a bland or lively backdrop to our lives? In my own practice, I use projectors of monochromatic light for highly specific color information. Each hue is absolutely pure, as opposed to the secondary mixtures achieved with polychromatic light, and this means that an infinite number of nuances can be produced in a seamless sequence. The narrow-band colors are projected into either a spherical dome or a visor, so all external cues of size and perspective are removed to make the inner space look infinite. (A planetarium is built on similar principles.) We call this a Ganzfeld (German for "whole-field") effect. The visual experience is similar to being suspended in a floating tank, and the hypnotic effect is very pronounced. In my own and other practices, light projectors are mainly used for a form of nonverbal psychotherapy.

Syntonics

The American optometrist Harry Spitler started beaming colored light directly into the eyes of his patients in the 1920s and 1930s, and syntonics is now widespread in the US. The colored-light irradiation is administrated through a long, narrow tube to make the most of the relatively weak incandescent light source. Normal treatments are done with stable and flicker-free light, but, if necessary, pulsations can be added. The technique utilizes a combination of eight glass filters to achieve a fuller range of intermediate hues. Syntonics is quite successful for treating visual problems in connection with head trauma.

Spectro-Chrome

The Indian engineer Dinshah Ghadiali treated plague victims in Bombay with colored beams emitted by an ordinary cinema projector. He later migrated to the US and expanded his light treatment to include fine glass filters capable of producing twelve rainbow hues. The method is now known as Spectro-Chrome. Colors are projected directly onto the naked skin in a system of separate body zones corresponding to the nervous system. For optimal effect, the irradiation or tonation alternates between complementary colors of high contrast.

Sensora

The Canadian physicist Anadi Martel has built an impressive multicolored system for projections on a large curved screen specially adapted to suit both the central and peripheral parts of the retina. His system is similar to a three-dimensional cinema and uses five LEDs pulsating in slowly modulated rhythms. The outcome is a color flow of great beauty and complexity combined with harmonizing music and integrated tactile stimulation. Spectators are seated on a vibrating settee that resonates in sync with the color modulations. Martel has also devised a semitransparent plastic globe that emits rotating polychromatic light in full surround. The sphere pulsates in tranquil color rhythms that never repeat themselves and run either by automatic program or by swiping your hand. The sphere radiates a pleasant glow with fascinating aesthetic and therapeutic qualities.

Eyelid irradiation

The German doctor Alexander Wunsch has developed a special method of phototherapy whereby colored light is beamed into the eyes through closed eyelids. The transmitted light will, of course, shift toward red, but offers a very soothing treatment that immediately reduces the risk of optic overload. A practical handheld pocket lamp with durable batteries provides absolutely flicker-free colored light suitable for home treatment of the chest, face, and eyes. Wunsch has also expanded the Spectro-Chrome method with a set of colored plastic spectacles in twelve highly saturated tones. Wearing these glasses is an exceptionally easy way of feeding colored light into the eyes and brain. It also incorporates a pleasant aspect of play, which is important when working with children.

Linear light

At Monocrom we have developed a special reading lamp designed to alleviate visual dyslexia. In this lamp, green LED light is modified through acrylic gratings, with parallel green stripes beamed onto the page to be read. These light lines help by suppressing the chaotic saccadic eye movements that are thought to be part of dyslexia.

Seeing the truth

As you can imagine, people respond in many ways to light therapy, but their responses tend to follow a similar pattern. Elation at being able to see pure color is often followed by an emotional high at the beauty of these true colors. However, often people will report pimples on the face, an upset tummy, or a snotty nose after treatment, all of which are normal, as precise and laser-like light will affect the living blood and rapidly multiply the amount of lymphocytes (see page 159). The vigorous detox process may also involve a cleansing of inner personal emotions, and we'll need to sleep well to recover. I have often found clients reporting vivid dreams after light treatment, and life changes, big and small, are not uncommon. It has also been my experience that my clients' intellectual performance has sharpened due to this photonic shot, and light therapy can be an excellent pre-exam boost. Many of my clients have had monochromatic light before exams, and their initial tiredness has abated.

MORE THERAPEUTIC COLOR

There seems to be no end to the fascinating effects of natural light and color, as we can see from the following potpourri of interesting insights.

Solarization

By drinking clear water, we continually replenish our bodies with precious liquid, but water is much more than a thirst-quencher: It is an optically active medium. This means that when irradiated with light, its electromagnetic arrangement will change: It has become solarized.

One of the most important effects of sunlight on water is well documented. UV destroys the DNA linkages in microorganisms, thus preventing them from reproducing and rendering them harmless. Solarized water is therefore safe to drink. The simplest way to solarize water is to place a glass of water in the sun. More sophisticated versions involve a colored glass or bottle. Green is commonly used for beer bottles to prevent rogue fermentation. Blue is used to prevent essential oils from deteriorating. Milk in brown bottles or cartons will take longer to go sour. This practice can be extended into your own daily health care. Pour good-quality water into a clear glass bottle, wrap a colored plastic filter around it, and place it in a sunny spot for two hours. Notice the difference in taste—mineral, salty, sweet, or bitter? Different-colored filters will impart different qualities to the water, and you will soon learn what benefits you.

Blue lavatories

In the 1990s, many big cities installed deep blue illumination in their public lavatories. The visual impact was surreal, but the intention was humanitarian. Any blue object would turn invisible under blue light and would be impossible to localize. Drug addicts could, therefore, no longer find their veins.

Prison life

Correctional institutions in Sweden have recently started to assimilate new design principles founded on the Dutch "Snoezelen" model, which has seen light and color used in multisensory environments for a number of years. The forensic psychiatric clinic in Växjö inaugurated a new pavilion in 2007 to serve severely troubled clients. Project manager Elisabet Hellgren developed a completely new interior based on artistic ideas aimed at creating an environment that emphasized safety and tranquility, both for employees and inmates. Instead of the traditional solitary confinement cells with restraining straps, she arranged softly padded rooms with music and harmonious color projections.

Operating theaters

In 2005, the Danish surgeon Jesper Durup installed color-changing light tubes in the operating theaters of Odense Hospital, Denmark. Soft chromatic light washes would partly replace the traditional white operating light that was decidedly monotonous and hard on the eyes. Ergonomic light colors would soothe the eyes of surgeons and nurses—possible because computerized operations demanded lower levels of illumination to avoid fading the monitors. The gentle color backgrounds would calm nervous patients before they received anesthesia and they would be less disoriented when waking up from narcosis. Full-power white spotlight was still necessary for open surgery given all the intricate maneuvers involved. Surgeons in the Catharina Hospital Eindhoven in the Netherlands have also operated under soft disco light in tones of pink, orange, and turquoise following the installation of an "ambient lighting scheme" in the cardiovascular room, and patients in the MRI scanning room in the Marien Hospital in Hamburg found the procedure very much more relaxing with the introduction of colored light.

CASE STUDY ON COLOR THERAPY FROM MY OWN PRACTICE

On a dark and gloomy autumn day, a very young woman arrived for her first light treatment with me. Hiding her face in her hands, she nervously told me a story of her deep depression. She found the darkness of winter unbearable and, having dropped out of school, was spending days lying in bed, curtains drawn. She had deep-seated fears that she might actually be going insane, and that other people could see the misery on her face. She was self-conscious about needing help and begged me not to tell anyone about her visits.

As I do for all my clients, I gave her the choice of colored lights, and she chose a mixture of bright pastel tints, of the kind that would be seen in springtime. She strongly rejected all blues, in particular hues of deep navy, as is often the case with clients suffering from winter depression. She scanned the colors impulsively and quickly, not stopping to contemplate any particular color selection. This free-flowing color strategy was used in all the following treatments.

After two sessions, she began to notice the difference, feeling a surge of happiness and energy. She cleaned up her messy bedroom and, as the light doses went on, began to experience an interest in running, which gave her a sense of freedom and self-confidence. Also, her now-regular exposure to sunlight stabilized her body clock and she would no longer lie in bed all day long. Her work life also began to improve; she sought training through a youth center and, after a hesitant start, turned out to be accurate and reliable at work and felt a sense of proud accomplishment. Then followed an expansive phase, where she joined her sister on a holiday trip to Spain. The light boost of Mediterranean sun was truly a boon, and she marveled at the thrill of different cultures. Sport and fitness became increasingly important, combined with an interest in massage and natural health, and she took up her studies again so she could work in this area.

When winter came around again, she found that occasional light doses were still needed to ward off depressive lapses, but her sessions became more and more infrequent as the winter blues receded. Interestingly, at her last light session with me, she flew through the colors of the spectrum at speed, but with one noticeable difference: Deep blue tones were no longer excluded. Her fear of darkness was gone.

GLOSSARY

Optical terms such as those in this glossary are frequently used in the world of lighting design and what we call "photonic engineering." According to the International Year of Light 2015, "*Photonics* is the science and technology of generating, controlling, and detecting photons, which are particles of light." Of course, you don't need an intimate knowledge of photonics in daily life, but some of the terms in this brave new world may pique your curiosity and comprehending them will be of practical benefit, as you'll understand the language of lighting designers and have a fair idea of what the technical labels mean. And you will not be fooled by misleading advertising campaigns. This glossary also provides definitions for other scientific terms that you'll have come across in the book.

Amplitude Indicates the magnitude of the oscillations in a continuous light wave. It is measured as the height of the crests and depth of the troughs. The square of the amplitude corresponds to the power or intensity of a beam. This value shows the quantity or volume of light available.

Ballast An electrical ballast is a device constructed to reduce the current in an electric circuit, which would otherwise rise to destructive levels. Many modern lamps have this included as a compact driving unit. Common examples are the inductive ballasts used in tubes to limit the pulsating current through the tube.

Bandwidth A measure to indicate the color precision of a mono-chromatic light wave. A broad bandwidth denotes a large spread of color with low saturation and lack of sharpness. A narrow bandwidth corresponds to restricted light movements with high saturation and full clarity of color. This value is typically in the range of some nanometers and measured in the middle of the wave.

Chronobiology Comes from the Greek *chronos*, meaning "time," and *biology*, meaning "the study of life." Chronobiology examines the cyclical processes of all living things and their interaction with solar and lunar rhythms.

Circadian Relates to physical and mental processes that happen over a twenty-four-hour period, for example, sleeping and waking, both of which are affected by light. You will have come across the term *biological clock*—this refers to the molecular timing device inside living organisms, from humans to bats to mice. This synchronizes our circadian rhythms so that certain biological processes happen at particular times of the day.

Coherence Vibratory patterns where all the waves join and reinforce each other in exactly the same phase or rhythm. All crests and troughs are in sync to precisely match the others, just like marching soldiers. Coherent light is generally produced by lasers, but many reflecting cavities can also generate it. In ordinary light, the wave patterns are randomly out of phase, even if each one may be monochromatic. Incoherent light is chaotic, and most of the vibratory energy cancels itself.

Color rendering index (CRI) A scale indicating the ability of an artificial light to represent colors faithfully compared to an "ideal" source, such as daylight. This is measured on a scale from 0 to 100. CRI is gradually being replaced by a new system, known as TM-30-15, which will become the new standard.

Color temperature Correlates the color of the emitted light with the temperature of its source. A low-temperature body radiates low energy in long wavelengths and is seen as reddish. A high-temperature body radiates high energy in short wavelengths and is perceived as bluish.

Daylight A loosely defined term for the strong white light radiating around midday. It is actually a mixture of two luminous components: direct sunlight with all its multiple surface reflections and scatterings, plus ambient background radiation from the blue sky.

Dichroic filter Di-layers, or double layers, of reflective coating, where light waves can bounce back and forth to reinforce and enhance each other. The color purity of dichroic filters is much higher than that of conventional plastic gels. Examples of dichroic filters are commonly seen in shiny metallic sunglasses.

Discharge This term turns up in the phrase "gas discharge lamps." These can be found in fluorescent light tubes and energy-saving lamps. Conductive gases are enclosed in a sealed tube and ignited by electrodes placed at the ends. Short electric pulses will make the gas glow in the ultraviolet range. Phosphorous compounds line the inside of the glass tube to modify the emitted radiation into whitish light.

Energy The energy in a light beam is directly proportional to the frequency of its waves. High-frequency and short waves always equal high optical energy levels. X-rays and ultraviolet are common examples of energy-rich radiation. Slow frequencies correspond to low energies and include infrared and microwaves.

Fiber optics An "optical fiber" is a transparent strand of glass or plastic. In fiber optics, these thin transparent threads can transport light like water through a hose to illuminate distant and hidden objects. The light is reflected off the insides of the shiny surfaces of glass or plastic. Optical fibers are used in computer-guided surgery, but also for advanced lighting design and telecommunication. Some natural fibers such as silk can also channel light.

Filter A transparent medium that absorbs certain wavelengths of light and lets others pass. A filter will always reduce the amount of incoming light and the transmitted remainder is often colored. Exceptions include colorless UV filters or IR screens. Common examples are plastic gels, tinted sunglasses, and colored liquids such as dyes.

Frequency The number of cycles per second in an oscillating wave. It is mathematically expressed as hertz (Hz). Audible sound typically lies at 1,000Hz or 1kHz. The frequency of visible light is much higher and lies in the magnitude of 10^{15}Hz. This gigantic and impractical number is seldom used, and light frequencies are often transcribed into nanometer (nm) wavelengths.

Hologram A microscopic rippled coating or photographic emulsion on a substrate of glass, plastic, or metal. It has a rippled micro surface, and like the surface of undulating water it will focus light in many points and patterns. It can either transmit or reflect the incoming beams. Some transmission holograms can focus the light into three-dimensional images. They are all produced using laser sources; common examples are found in modern passports or on banknotes.

Incandescence The light emitted by bodies when heated to sufficiently high temperatures. This could be the red-hot iron in a blacksmith's forge or even a cluster of stars. Emission of incandescent light is a special case of thermal radiation known as blackbody radiation, or Planck radiation. Incandescent light sources include a metal wire that is electrically heated until it emits a continuous light flow. Common examples are standard light bulbs and halogen lamps.

Infrared A form of electromagnetic radiation of a particular wavelength, between 700nm and 1mm, just beyond the red end of the rainbow. Common uses for infrared include TV remote controls, closed-circuit television, and infrared saunas.

Interference The mutual interaction of wave patterns between adjacent light beams. In creative interference, crests and troughs enhance each other and create beautiful light phenomena. In destructive interference, the crests and troughs cancel each other and give only darkness. Common examples are the colored light ripples in soap bubbles and rainbows.

Ionization An isolated atom is always electrically neutral, with an equal number of electrons and protons in balance. In ionized light sources, outer electrons are removed and the remaining atom becomes positively charged and conducts electricity. The removal can happen through light, electricity, or heat.

Kelvin A unit of temperature measurement, used along with Fahrenheit and Celsius, named after the Belfast inventor William Thompson, Lord Kelvin. "Absolute zero" on the Kelvin scale refers to the temperature at which molecules would stop moving, moving up incrementally to boiling point. The color temperature of lights is measured in kelvin (K).

Laser An acronym for "light amplification by stimulated emission of radiation." Invented in 1960, it is an artificial light source with exceptional precision and light density. Electrical discharges pump light waves to oscillate back and forth inside a resonating amplifying medium. The emitted beams have a very high radiant power and can be used to cut steel. Laser light is coherent, polarized, and monochromatic. Common examples are found in laser pointers and supermarket cash tills.

LED An acronym for "light-emitting diode." A very compact diode made from two semiconducting materials sandwiched together. An electric current is applied and electrons in the semiconductors are forced to recombine with their positive opposites or holes. They mutually annihilate each other in a superefficient release of light. High output and small size plus extremely long life span make LED light interesting for energy-saving. Common examples are found in traffic lights and pocket flashlights.

Lens A lenticular body of transparent material such as glass, quartz, or plastic. Parallel light beams passing a convex or curved lens will converge into a focal point, via what you will know as a magnifying glass. You might also know that they can collect sunrays to ignite fire. A concave or hollow lens will scatter and divert incoming rays. It will diminish all images and cannot focus light. Modern lenses are often made of plastic to transmit ultraviolet radiation. The human eye contains an organic lens of transparent protein crystals.

Fresnel lens A flattened version of a classical lens, with a surface broken up into concentric rings of narrow ridges. This makes it much thinner and lighter than a conventional full-bodied lens. It can be made out of glass or plastic. Large Fresnel lenses molded out of transparent plastic are quite inexpensive. Common examples are seen in the rear windows of buses.

Lighting supplier This refers to any source of lighting, from your home superstore to a hardware store, online supplier, or even supermarket.

Liquid crystal A semiliquid gel with transparent oblong molecules arranged in orderly and often parallel structures. Incident light beams prefer to travel along the longitudinal axis of the crystal-like formations. The asymmetric molecules are sensitive to electric stimulation and can be manipulated to move. Common examples are computer screens and biological membrane tissues.

Luminescence A luminous radiation emitted by bodies at low temperatures. Two molecules with high chemical energy combine and spontaneously give off light. One is typically a pigment and the other is an enzyme. Luminescence is mostly found in biological systems and used for animal communication. Common examples are the green lights of fireflies and glowworms.

Lux/lumens Measurements of light intensity, with one lux roughly comparing to the illumination provided by a full moon. A lumen is a standardized unit of measurement for the total amount of light produced by a light source, such as a lamp. One lux is defined as being equivalent to one lumen spread over an area of one square meter.

Lymphocytes These are part of a family of white blood cells. Lymphocytes are produced in the lymph nodes and act as natural body guards. They systematically kill and scavenge harmful biological invaders.

Mirror Thin layers of silver or aluminum deposited on a glass surface. The delicate shiny foils are often hidden on the back for better protection. High-quality astronomy mirrors have the metal film on the front to avoid double reflections. Mirrors can be curved or flat. A plane mirror will not distort the reflected light, while a concave or hollow mirror will collect incoming rays into a point of focus and produce a magnified image. The light reflected from a convex mirror is dissipated in all directions and these mirrors have no focus; the image on their reflecting surface will look smaller than real life.

Monochromatic A Greek word meaning "one-colored," as opposed to polychromatic or many-colored. The wave packages of monochromatic light beams have exactly the same frequency where distances between all peaks and troughs are identical. These lights are of intense appearance, and the single color projected will be of maximal saturation. Common examples are scarabs and butterflies.

OLED Acronym for "organic light-emitting diode." Thin sheets of organic plastic polymers are placed between two slim electrical conductors. An external current is applied and the electrostatic plastics then become luminous and generate a white light with reasonable spectral qualities. Common examples are seen in mobile phones and computer screens.

Phosphorescence A combination process similar to luminescence, in which a photoactive chemical absorbs incoming light and then ejects it but with reemission much delayed. Common examples are clock dials and paints that glow in the dark.

Photon A minuscule and massless elemental particle traveling at the speed of light in a vacuum. It is electrically neutral and extremely stable and does not spontaneously decay. Photons of sufficient energy can knock outer electrons into excited orbits and enable them to participate in photobiological reactions. The photon model describes a physical particle, but this is only a partial illustration of light. Light therapy and photobiology make use of the photon model.

Photonic crystal A multidimensional and highly complex crystal structure, which selectively refracts incoming rays. It can be made naturally from intricate protein scales or artificially constructed from glass or plastic. When radiated, it emits light that is often highly monochromatic. Well-known examples are shimmering butterfly wings and opals.

Plasma A strongly heated and ionized gas, where the atoms have been stripped of electrons. Burning plasma spontaneously emits light. It is electrically conductive and therefore affected by external electric or magnetic fields. Artificial plasma lights can be directed and manipulated. Common examples are carbon arc lights and the solar corona.

Polarized light Contains two vibrating components that oscillate at right angles to each other. One is magnetic and one is electric, and the pair normally rotate in all possible directions. When this rotating bundle is reflected or filtered it loses this freedom and becomes polarized. It will now vibrate in one plane only. Common examples are moonlight and shimmering asphalt surfaces.

Polychromatic Light beams composed of waves with different frequencies or colors. The different colors compete and cancel each other out. In cases of high randomization the canceling is total and the final color will appear to be faded or completely white. This is the most normal form of light. Common examples are sunlight and white artificial light.

Prism A transparent, geometric body of glass, plastic, crystal, or ice with a varying number of rectilinear sides. In triangular prisms the light will always deviate toward the base. A common example is the three-sided prism, as once used in Newton's color experiment.

Semiconducting diodes A semiconductor is a material that reacts to an electrical current, with greater resistance in one direction than in another.

Spectrum The visible spectrum is also referred to as the "optical window" and contains the full rainbow sequence. Sometimes infrared and ultraviolet are included. The part we can see is just a tiny element of the much greater electromagnetic spectrum, which extends all the way from cosmic rays to sonic waves. A common example of a visible spectrum is the rainbow.

Suprachiasmatic nucleus (SCN) This group of thousands of neurons is found in the hypothalamus and is sometimes referred to as the "master clock," keeping all the other biological processes in sync.

Transmission The amount of light that can freely pass through an optical medium. It indicates the percentage of the incident white light (incoming unfiltered light) that will pass through the medium. Sometimes the term is used to indicate the degree of transparency. The opposite property of transparent is opaque.

Watt A unit of power named after James Watt, the British scientist, which describes the amount of electric power that it produces or uses.

Wave A vibratory oscillation in a medium. Light can partly be illustrated as electromagnetic disturbances of the vacuum field. Light waves vibrate sideways and are described as *transverse*, as opposed to the longitudinal waves of sound. Common examples of waves are seen in moving skipping ropes and in ripples on the surface of a pond.

FURTHER READING

Not all of these texts will be available to the general reader, but I have found them to be useful references for my own practice.

BOOKS

Babbitt, E. *The Principles of Light and Color*. New York: Babbitt & Co., 1878.

Bates, W. *Perfect Sight Without Glasses*. New York: Burr, 1920.

Baxter, D. *Therapeutic Lasers*. London: Churchill Livingstone, 1994.

Bernhard, O. *Light Treatment in Surgery*. London: Arnold, 1926.

Boyce, P. *Human Factors in Lighting*. London: Taylor & Francis, 2003.

Breiling, B., ed. *Light Years Ahead*. Tiburon, CA: LYA Publishing, 1996.

Chang, J., et al., eds. *Biophotons*. Dordrecht, Netherlands: Kluwer Academic Publishers, 1998.

Clausen, H. *Light & Communication*. Hillerød, Denmark: Meldorf Hansen, 2009.

Coghill, R. *The Healing Energies of Light*. London: Gaia, 2000.

Dillon, K. *Healing Photons*. Washington, DC: Scientia Press, 1998.

Dinshah, D. *Let There Be Light*. Málaga, Spain: Dinshah Society, 1985.

Downing, D. *Daylight Robbery*. London: Arrow, 1988.

Ensminger, P. *Life Under the Sun*. New Haven, CT: Yale University Press, 2001.

Finsen, N. *Phototherapy*. London: Arnold, 1901.

Gimbel, T. *Healing with Color & Light*. New York: Simon & Schuster, 1994.

Grossweiner, L. *The Science of Phototherapy: An Introduction*. Dordrecht, Netherlands: Springer, 2005.

Hobday, R. *The Healing Sun*. Findhorn, Scotland: Findhorn Press, 1999.

———. *The Light Revolution*. Findhorn, Scotland: Findhorn Press, 2006.

Holick, M. *The UV Advantage*. New York: ibooks, 2003.

Howat, D. *Elements of Chromotherapy*. London: Actinic Press, 1938.

Karu, T. *Ten Lectures on Basic Science of Laser Therapy*. Grängesberg, Sweden: Prima Books, 2007.

Kime, Z. *Sunlight*. Penryn, UK: World Health, 1980.

Krusen, F. *Light Therapy*. New York: Hoeber, 1937.

le Grand, Y. *An Introduction to Photobiology*. London: Faber & Faber, 1970.

Liberman, J. *Light: Medicine of the Future*. Santa Fe, NM: Bear & Company, 1991.

Mandel, P. *The Practical Compendium of Colorpuncture*. Bruchsal, Germany: Energetik Verlag, 1986.

Mighall, R. *Sunshine*. London: John Murray, 2008.

Millar, R., and Free, E. *Sunrays and Health*. New York: McBride, 1929.

Mizon, B. *Light Pollution*. London: Springer, 2002.

Ott, J. *Health and Light*. Columbus, OH: Ariel Press, 1973.

Pöntinen, P. *Low Level Laser Therapy as a Medical Treatment Modality*. Tampere, Finland: Art Urpo, 1992.

Regan, J., and Parrish, J. *The Science of Photomedicine*. New York: Plenum Press, 1982.

Rollier, A. *Heliotherapy*. London: Hodder & Stoughton, 1923.

Rosenthal, N., and Blehar, M. *Seasonal Affective Disorders and Phototherapy*. New York: Guilford Press, 1989.

Senger, H., ed. *Blue Light Effects in Biological Systems*. Berlin: Springer, 1984.

Spitler, H. *The Syntonic Principle*. Eaton, OH: College of Syntonic Optometry, 1990.

Stanway, P. *Life Light*. London: Kyle Cathie, 2001.

Tunér, J., and Hode, L. *The New Laser Therapy Handbook*. Grängesberg, Sweden: Prima Books, 2010.

ARTICLES AND REPORTS

Abizaid, A., et al. "Direct Visual and Circadian Pathways Target Neuroendocrine Cells in Primates." *European Journal of Neuroscience* 20, no. 10 (December 2004): 2767–76.

Barrett, D., and Gonzalez-Lima, F. "Transcranial Infrared Laser Stimulation Produces Beneficial Cognitive and Emotional Effects in Humans." *Neuroscience* 230 (2013): 13–23.

Berson, D., et al. "Phototransduction by Retinal Ganglion Cells That Set the Circadian Clock." *Science* 295, no. 5557 (February 8, 2002): 1070–73.

Bourgin, P., and Hubbard, J. "Alerting or Somnogenic Light: Pick Your Color." *Public Library of Science* 14, no. 8 (August 15, 2016): 1–8.

Bullough, J. "The Blue-Light Hazard: A Review." *Journal of the Illuminating Engineering Society* 29, no. 2 (Summer 2000): 6–14.

Casal, J., and Yanovsky, M. "Regulation of Gene Expression by Light." *International Journal of Developmental Biology* 49, nos. 5–6 (2005): 501–11.

Dewan, E., et al. "Effects of Photic Stimulation on the Human Menstrual Cycle." *Photochemistry and Photobiology* 27, no. 5 (May 1978): 581–85.

Fonken, L., et al. "Light at Night Increases Body Mass by Shifting the Time of Food Intake." *Proceedings of the National Academy of Sciences USA* 107, no. 43 (October 26, 2010): 18664–69.

Foster, R., and Roenneberg, T. "Human Responses to the Geophysical Daily, Annual and Lunar Cycles." *Current Biology* 18, no. 17 (September 9, 2008): R784–R794.

Heshong, L., et al. *Windows and Offices: A Study of Office Worker Performance and the Indoor Environment.* Sacramento, CA: California Energy Commission, 2003, 5–11.

Hill, R., and Barton, R. "Red Enhances Human Performance in Contests." *Nature* 435 (May 19, 2005): 293.

Kohsaka, M., et al. "Effects of Bright Light Exposure on Heart Rate Variability During Sleep in Young Women." *Psychiatry and Clinical Neurosciences* 55 (2001): 283–84.

Küller, R., and Laike, T. "The Impact of Flicker from Fluorescent Lighting on Well-Being, Performance and Physiological Arousal." *Ergonomics* 41, no. 4 (April 1998): 433–47.

Land, M. "Motion and Vision: Why Animals Move Their Eyes." *Journal of Comparative Physiology* 185, no. 4 (October 1999): 341–52.

Partonen, T., and Lönnqvist, J. "Bright Light Improves Vitality and Alleviates Distress in Healthy People." *Journal of Affective Disorders* 57, nos. 1–3 (January–March 2000): 55–61.

Roelandts, R. "A New Light on Niels Finsen, a Century After His Nobel Prize." *Photodermatology, Photoimmunology & Photomedicine* 21, no. 3 (June 2005): 115–17.

Rybnikova, N., et al. "Artificial Light at Night (ALAN) and Breast Cancer Incidence Worldwide: A Revisit of Earlier Findings with Analysis of Current Trends." *Chronobiology International* 32, no. 6 (2015): 757–73.

Schiffer, F., et al. "Psychological Benefits 2 and 4 Weeks After a Single Treatment with Near Infrared Light to the Forehead: A Pilot Study of 10 Patients with Major Depression and Anxiety." *Behavioural and Brain Functions* 5 (2009): 46.

Whelan, H., et al. "Effect of Nasa Light-Emitting Diode Irradiation on Wound Healing." *Journal of Clinical Medicine & Surgery* 19, no. 6 (December 2001): 305–14.

USEFUL LINKS

www.aahlight.com/red-light-therapy

www.bioptron.com/products/bioptron-2.aspx

www.bupa.co.uk/health-information/directory/l/light-therapy

www.collegeofsyntonicoptometry.com

www.color-institute.com

www.darksky.org

www.enchroma.com

www.energyandvibration.com/light.htm

www.inlightmedical.com

www.int.aesthetic.lutronic.com/intl/professionals/treatments/light
  -therapy
www.international-light-association.org
www.laser.nu
www.lightforfitness.com
www.lighttherapydevice.com
www.lrc.rpi.edu
www.lumasoothe.com
www.lumie.com
www.mayoclinic.org
www.medscape.com/viewarticle/854857
www.monocrom.se
www.neutrogena.com/category/acne/light+therapy+acne+mask.do
www.philips.co.uk/shop/personalcare/dermatology/c/PSORIASIS
  _TREATMENT_SU
www.photonichealth.com
www.pld-alliance.org
www.psoriasis.org/about-psoriasis/treatments/phototherapy
www.psychologytoday.com/blog/sleepless-in-america/201101/light
  -therapy
www.redlightman.com/light-therapy
www.sensora.com
www.sltbr.org
www.thedermreview.com/red-light-therapy
www.toptenreviews.com/health/wellness/best-light-therapy-lamps
www.verilux.com
www.vimeo.com/alexanderwunsch/videos
www.waltza.co.za
www.wikipedia.org/wiki/seasonal_affective_disorder
www.yogajournal.com

NOTES

1 R. J. Wells, J. R. Gionfriddo, T. B. Hackett, and S. V. Radecki, "Canine and Feline Emergency Room Visits and the Lunar Cycle: 11,940 Cases (1992–2002)," *Journal of the American Veterinary Medical Association* 231, no. 2 (July 15, 2007): 251–53.

2 L. Conti, "How Light Deprivation Causes Depression," *Scientific American*, August 1, 2008, www.scientificamerican.com/article /down-in-the-dark.

3 D. Cox, "The Science of SAD: Understanding the Causes of 'Winter Depression,'" *Guardian*, October 30, 2017, www.the guardian.com/lifeandstyle/2017/oct/30/sad-winter-depression -seasonal-affective-disorder.

4 K. P. Wright Jr., A. W. McHill, B. R. Birks, B. R. Griffin, T. Rusterholz, and E. D. Chinoy, "Entrainment of the Human Circadian Clock to the Natural Light-Dark Cycle," *Current Biology* 23, no. 16 (August 19, 2013): 1554–58, https://doi.org/10.1016 /j.cub.2013.06.039.

5 D. K. Randall, *Dreamland: Adventures in the Strange Science of Sleep* (New York: W. W. Norton & Co., 2013).

6 "Is Artificial Lighting Making Us Sick? New Evidence in Mice," *Science Daily*, July 14, 2016, www.sciencedaily.com/releases/2016 /07/160714134753.htm.

7 M. Halper, "Here Comes the Graphene LED Bulb," *Lux Review*, March 30, 2015, www.luxreview.com/article/2015/03/here-comes -the-graphene-led-bulb.

8 I. Sample, "Matter Will Be Created from Light Within a Year, Claim

Scientists," *Guardian*, May 18, 2014, www.theguardian.com/science/2014/may/18/matter-light-photons-electrons-positrons.

9   N. Bunnin and J. Yu, *The Blackwell Dictionary of Western Philosophy* (Hoboken, NJ: John Wiley & Sons, 2008).

10   "Vitamin D," NHS, last reviewed March 3, 2017, www.nhs.uk/conditions/vitamins-and-minerals/vitamin-d.

11   "Daylighting and Productivity," Heschong Mahone Group, accessed June 8, 2018, http://h-m-g.com/projects/daylighting/projects-PIER.htm.

12   "Daylighting Facts and Figures," Solatube Group, accessed June 8, 2018, www.solatube.com/sites/default/files/field/files/tech_resources/daylight-facts-figures-retail-sales.pdf.

13   C. Bergland, "Exposure to Natural Light Improves Workplace Performance," *Psychology Today*, June 5, 2013, www.psychologytoday.com/blog/the-athletes-way/201306/exposure-natural-light-improves-workplace-performance.

14   M. Dacke, D. E. Nilsson, C. H. Scholtz, M. Byrne, and E. J. Warrant, "Animal Behaviour: Insect Orientation to Polarized Moonlight," *Nature* 424, no. 33 (July 3, 2003), http://www.nature.com/articles/424033a.

15   C. Rastad, P. O. Sjödén, and J. Ulfberg, "High Prevalence of Self-Reported Winter Depression in a Swedish County," *Psychiatry and Clinical Neurosciences* 59, no. 6, (December 2005): 666–75.

16   C. Nierenberg, "The Weird Way Your Latitude May Affect Your Blood Pressure," *Live Science*, May 18, 2016, https://www.livescience.com/54789-latitude-may-affect-blood-pressure.html.

17   "Time for More Vitamin D," *Harvard Health Publishing*, September 2008, www.health.harvard.edu/staying-healthy/time-for-more-vitamin-d.

18   C. Milmo, "Not Just the Stuff of Legend: Famed Viking 'Sunstone' Did Exist, Believe Scientists," *Independent*, March 6, 2013, https://www.independent.co.uk/news/science/archaeology/not-just-the-stuff-of-legend-famed-viking-sunstone-did-exist-believe-scientists-8521522.html.

19 "How Do I Protect Myself from UV Rays?," American Cancer Society, last modified May 22, 2017, www.cancer.org/cancer/skin -cancer/prevention-and-early-detection/uv-protection.

20 J. McIntosh, "The Impact of Shift Work on Health," *Medical News Today*, January 11, 2016, www.medicalnewstoday.com/articles /288310.php.

21 M. Abrahams, "Strange but True: Science's Most Improbable Research," *Guardian*, August 18, 2012, www.theguardian .com/science/2012/aug/19/most-improbable-scientific-research -abrahams.

22 O. Al-Ghazawy, "The Growing Danger of Osteoporosis in the Arab World," *Nature Middle East*, November 29, 2011, https:// www.natureasia.com/en/nmiddleeast/article/10.1038/nmiddle east.2011.158.

23 "Color Temperature and Color Rendering Index Demystified," Tiffen, accessed June 6, 2018, http://lowel.tiffen.com/edu/color _temperature_and_rendering_demystified.

24 S. R. Lim, D. Kang, O. A. Ogunseitan, and J. M. Schoenung, "Potential Environmental Impacts of Light-Emitting Diodes (LEDs): Metallic Resources, Toxicity, and Hazardous Waste Clas- sification," *Environmental Science & Technology* 45, no. 1 (January 1, 2011): 320–27.

25 C. C. M. Kyba, T. Kuester, A. Sanchez de Miguel, K. Baugh, A. Jeshow, F. Holker, J. Bennie, C. D. Elvidge, K.J. Gaston, and L. Ganter, "Artificially Lit Surface of Earth at Night Increasing in Radiance and Extent," *Science Advances* 3, no. 11 (November 2017), http://advances.sciencemag.org/content/3/11/e1701528.full.

26 E. Zachos, "Too Much Light at Night Causes Spring to Come Early," *National Geographic*, June 28, 2016, https://news .nationalgeographic.com/2016/06/light-pollution-early-spring -budbursts.

27 D. Martin, "Douglas Leigh, the Man Who Lit Up Broadway, Dies at 92," *New York Times*, December 16, 1999, www.nytimes.com /learning/students/pop/articles/obit-d-leigh.html.

28 S. Higuchi, Y. Motohashi, L. Yang, and A. Maeda, "Effects of
    Playing a Computer Game Using a Bright Display on Presleep
    Physiological Variables, Sleep Latency, Slow Wave Sleep and REM
    Sleep," *Journal of Sleep Research* 14, no. 3 (September 2005): 267–
    73, https://doi.org/10.1111/j.1365-2869.2005.00463.x.

29 M. Dunbar and D. Melton, "The Lowdown on Blue Light:
    Good vs. Bad, and Its Connection to AMD," *Review of Optom-
    etry*, accessed February 2018, www.reviewofoptometry.com/ce
    /the-lowdown-on-blue-light-good-vs-bad-and-its-connection-to
    -amd-109744.

30 R. Steinbach, C. Perkins, L. Tompson, S. Johnson, B. Armstrong,
    J. Green, C. Grundy, P. Wilkinson, and P. Edwards, "The Effect
    of Reduced Street Lighting on Road Casualties and Crime in
    England and Wales: Controlled Interrupted Time Series Analysis,"
    Journal of Epidemiology & Community Health 69, no. 11 (Novem-
    ber 2015): 1118–24, http://dx.doi.org/10.1136/jech-2015-206012.

31 N. Rosenthal, "On the Frontiers of SAD: How Much Light Is
    Enough?," *Norman Rosenthal, MD* (blog), January 3, 2012, www
    .normanrosenthal.com/blog/2012/01/seasonal-affective-disorder
    -light-therap.

32 D. Berryman, "10 Tips for Buying SAD Lights," SAD.org.uk, Jan-
    uary 4, 2017, www.sad.org.uk/10-tips-buying-sad-lights.

33 "Niels Ryberg Finsen—Facts," The Nobel Prize, Nobel Media AB,
    accessed June 8, 2018, www.nobelprize.org/nobel_prizes/medicine
    /laureates/1903/finsen-facts.html.

34 J. Sequeira, "Seven Years' Experience of the Finsen Treatment," *The
    Lancet* 171, no. 4410 (March 17, 1908): 713–16.

35 R. Sexton, "Slip, Slop, Crack: The Vitamin D Crisis," *The Age*,
    December 9, 2007, www.theage.com.au/articles/2007/12/08
    /1196813083745.html.

36 According to research from M. Feelisch, B. Fernandez, A. Ham-
    ilton, N. N. Laing, J. M. C. Gallagher, D. E. Newby, R. Weller,
    "UVA Irradiation of Human Skin Vasodilates Arterial Vascula-

ture and Lowers Blood Pressure Independently of Nitric Oxide Synthase," *Journal of Investigative Dermatology*, December 8, 2015. Quoted in "Sunlight Might Be Good for Your Blood Pressure," by Steven Reinberg, WebMD, https://www.webmd.com/hyper tension-high-blood-pressure/news/20140120/sunlight-might-be -good-for-your-blood-pressure-study#.

37 "Here Comes the Sun to Lower Your Blood Pressure," News, University of Southampton, January 20, 2014, www.southampton .ac.uk/news/2014/01/20-the-sun-to-lower-your-blood-pressure .page.

38 Georgetown University Medical Center, "Sunlight Offers Surprise Benefit—It Energizes Infection Fighting T Cells," press release, December 20, 2016, https://gumc.georgetown.edu/news /sunlight-offers-surprise-benefit-it-energizes-infection-fighting -t-cells.

39 T. Oliver, "Top Cancer Doctor Says You SHOULD Have a Sunbed Session," *Daily Mail*, last modified January 24, 2009, www.dailymail.co.uk/health/article-1127175/Top-cancer-doctor -says-SHOULD-sunbed-session.html#ixzz55Hs5R6Wh.

40 "How Do I Get the Vitamin D My Body Needs?," Vitamin D Council, accessed June 8, 2018, www.vitamindcouncil.org /about-vitamin-d/how-do-i-get-the-vitamin-d-my-body-needs.

41 K. Young, "The Safe Guide to Buying and Using Sunscreen," *Telegraph*, May 27, 2016, www.telegraph.co.uk/beauty/skin/the-safe -guide-to-buying-and-using-sunscreen.

42 Ibid.

43 J. Stromberg, "A Hot Drink on a Hot Day Can Cool You Down," *Smithsonian*, July 10, 2012, www.smithsonianmag.com/science -nature/a-hot-drink-on-a-hot-day-can-cool-you-down-1338875.

44 M. James, "36 Mind Blowing Facts about Infrared Radiation (IR Rays)," June 25, 2017, www.infrared-light-therapy.com/infra red-radiation/.

45 G. D. Gale, P. J. Rothbart, and Y. Li, "Infrared Therapy for Chronic

Low Back Pain: A Randomized, Controlled Trial," *Pain Research and Management* 11, no. 3 (Autumn 2006): 193–96, www.ncbi.nlm.nih.gov/pmc/articles/PMC2539004/.

46 D. Pavliv and S. Wang, "Does Infrared Light Therapy Work for Weight Loss?," National Center for Health Research, accessed June 8, 2018, www.center4research.org/infrared-light-therapy-work-weight-loss.

47 J. H. Lee, M. R. Roh, and K. H. Lee, "Effects of Infrared Radiation on Skin Photo-Aging and Pigmentation," *Yonsei Medical Journal* 47, no. 4 (August 31, 2006): 485–90.

48 F. G. Oosterveld, J. J. Rasker, M. Floors, R. Landkroon, B. van Rennes, J. Zwijnenberg, M.A. van de Laar, and G. J. Koel, "Infrared Sauna in Patients with Rheumatoid Arthritis and Ankylosing Spondylitis," *Clinical Rheumatology* 28, no. 1 (January 2009): 29, https://doi.org/10.1007/s10067-008-0977-y.

49 J. Goldman, "Pupils Dilate or Expand in Response to Mere Thoughts of Light or Dark," *Scientific American*, March 1, 2014, www.scientificamerican.com/article/pupils-dilate-expand-respond-thought-light-dark.

50 X. La Canna, "Prince Harry 'May Need Binoculars' to Match 'Super Sight' of Indigenous NORFORCE Soldiers," ABC News, last modified April 8, 2105, www.abc.net.au/news/2015-04-08/prince-harry-may-struggle-to-keep-up-with-aboriginal-super-sight/6378066.

51 N. Collins, "Time Spent Outdoors Linked to Better Eyesight," *Telegraph*, October 24, 2011, www.telegraph.co.uk/news/health/children/8846020/Time-spent-outdoors-linked-to-better-eyesight.html.

52 J. Maas, R. A. Verheij, S. de Vries, P. Spreeuwenberg, F. G. Schellevis, and P. P. Groenewegen, "Morbidity Is Related to a Green Living Environment," *Journal of Epidemiology & Community Health* 63, no. 12 (December 2009): 967–73, doi: 10.1136/jech.2008.079038.

53 "Nature Makes Us More Caring, Study Says," University of Roch-

ester, September 30, 2009, www.rochester.edu/news/show.php?id
=3450.

54 A. Perez, "AD Classics: The Farnsworth House / Mies van der
Rohe," *Arch Daily*, May 13, 2010, www.archdaily.com/59719
/ad-classics-the-farnsworth-house-mies-van-der-rohe.

55 "Transforming the Lighting Landscape," US Department of
Energy, last modified November 1, 2016, www.lightingprize.org.

56 C. Cleary, "Almost Half of Food in Irish Shopping Baskets Is
Ultra-Processed," *Irish Times*, February 7, 2018, www.irishtimes
.com/life-and-style/food-and-drink/almost-half-of-food-in-irish
-shopping-baskets-is-ultra-processed-1.3382342.

57 European Food Safety Authority, *Chemicals in Food 2016: Over-
view of Selected Data Collection*, 2016, www.efsa.europa.eu/sites
/default/files/corporate_publications/files/161215chemicalsin
foodreport.pdf.

58 T. H. Wakamatsu, M. Dogru, and K. Tsubota, "Tearful Rela-
tions: Oxidative Stress, Inflammation and Eye Diseases," *Arquivos
Brasileirosde Oftalmologia* 71, no. 6 (November/December 2008):
72–79, http://dx.doi.org/10.1590/S0004-27492008000700015.

59 M. Friedman, S. O. Byers, and R. H. Rosenman, "Effect of Unsat-
urated Fats upon Lipemia and Conjunctival Circulation: A Study of
Coronary-Prone (Pattern A) Men," *Journal of the American Medical
Association* 193, no. 11 (September 13, 1965): 882–86.

60 M. C. Moore, M. A. Guzman, P. E. Schilling, and J. P. Strong,
"Dietary-Atherosclerosis Study on Deceased Persons," *Journal of the
American Dietetic Association* 79, no. 6 (December 1981): 668–72.

61 "How Can I Reduce My Sugar Intake?," BBC, accessed June 8,
2018, www.bbc.co.uk/guides/ztfpn39#z9ctpv4.

62 L. Copeland, "Where Men See White, Women See Ecru," *Smithsonian*, March 2013, www.smithsonianmag.com/science-nature
/where-men-see-white-women-see-ecru-22540446.

63 "Facts About Color Blindness," National Eye Institute, last modified February 2015, www.nei.nih.gov/health/color_blindness/facts
_about.

64 "Blinded by the Night," *Harvard Health Publishing*, June 2007, www.health.harvard.edu/diseases-and-conditions/blinded-by-the -night.

65 K. Menju, "The Effect of Visible Light upon the Secretion of Milk," *Japanese Journal of Obstetrics and Gynaecology* 23, no. 3 (1940):130–40.

INDEX